AUG 2 8 2012

ADVANCED–EXPERT SECOND EDITION

D1706348

DISCARD

SKI AND SNOWBOARD GUIDE TO
WHISTLER BLACKCOMB

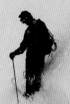

Distributed by
Gordon Soules Book Publishers Ltd.
1359 Ambleside Lane,
West Vancouver, BC, Canada V7T 2Y9
books@gordonsoules.com
604-922-6588 Fax: 604-922-6574

SKI & SNOWBOARD GUIDE TO WHISTLER BLACKCOMB

QUICKDRAW
PUBLICATIONS

POSTAL ADDRESS
PO Box 5313
Squamish, BC V8B 0C2
Canada

CONTACT US
(604) 892-9271
info@quickdrawpublications.com

Quickdraw Publications is constantly expanding our range of guidebooks. If you have a manuscript or an idea for a book, please get in touch.

Designed and typeset in Canada; printed and bound in China.

ADVANCED–EXPERT SECOND EDITION

INTERNATIONAL STANDARD BOOK NUMBER
ISBN 978-0-9877796-0-1

AUTHORS
Brian Finestone & Kevin Hodder

PHOTOGRAPHY
All photographs by Brian Finestone unless otherwise noted. Cover photo: Duncan Mackenzie deep in Whistler Bowl. Page one photo: Kevin Labatte committed to the beast above Road Runner. This page: Tony Sittlinger scoping the avalanche hazard in Blackcomb Bowl.

Disclaimer

READ THIS BEFORE YOU USE THIS BOOK!

Warning: Skiing and snowboarding are sports which involve inherent risks. Participating in these sports may result in injury or death.

This guidebook is intended to be used by expert skiers and snowboarders only. The terrain described within is dangerous and requires a high level of experience to negotiate.

This guidebook is a compilation of information from several sources. As a result the authors cannot confirm the accuracy of any specific detail. Difficulty ratings are subjective and may vary depending on your own personal experience and the conditions on the mountain. There may be misinformation in regards to run description, condition, or difficulty.

This guidebook does not give the user the right to access any terrain described within. The ski patrol may limit access to any part of the mountain at any time or change the ski area boundaries at any time. It is your responsibility to adhere to all closures.

This guidebook is not a substitute for experience and proper judgment. Your use of this book indicates your assumption of the risk that it may contain errors and is an acknowledgement of your own sole responsibility for your safety.

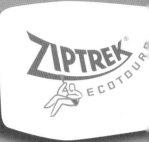

Breathtaking!
eco-exhilaration™

DISCLAIMER 3

INTRODUCTION 6
About This Book 8
How to Use This Book 8
Furthering Your Enjoyment 10
2010 Winter Olympics 12
Avoiding Lineups 14
Parking 15
On Hill Signage 16
Code of Conduct 18
Safety 18
Avalanche Control 21
Hazards 24
Backcountry Access 26
Weather 28

WHISTLER MOUNTAIN 34
Ski Area Overview 36
1. Roundhouse Zone West 38
2. Roundhouse Zone East 44
3. The Lower Glades 48
4. T-Bar Zone 52
5. Little Whistler 58
6. Harmony Ridge 60
7. Sun Bowl Zone 64
8. Symphony Zone 70
9. Flute 77
10. Glacier Bowl 82
11. Whistler Bowl 84
12. Lower Peak Chair Zone 88
13. West Ridge 92
14. West Bowl 96
15. Peak to Creek 100

PEAK 2 PEAK 104

BLACKCOMB MOUNTAIN 108
Ski Area Overview 110
1. Solar Coaster Zone 112
2. Jersey Cream Bowl 116
3. Lakeside Bowl 120
4. Blackcomb Glacier 122
5. Gemstone Bowls 128
6. Swiss Cheese 138
7. Secret Bowl 140

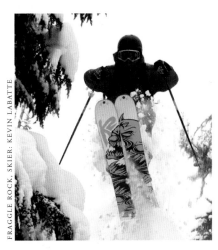

FRAGGLE ROCK, SKIER: KEVIN LABATTE

8. Crystal Traverse 144
9. Grey Zone and Opal Bowl 146
10. Crystal Chair Zone 148
11. Chainsaw Ridge 153
12. Horstman Peak 159

MOUNTAIN EXTRAS 162
Terrain Parks 164
Link-ups 170
The Groomed Runs 172
Don't Miss List 174
Events 176
Index 178
Acknowledgements 182
About the Authors 184

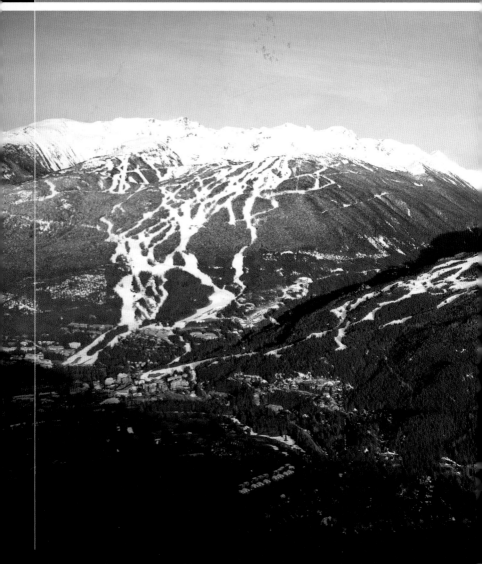

INTRODUCTION

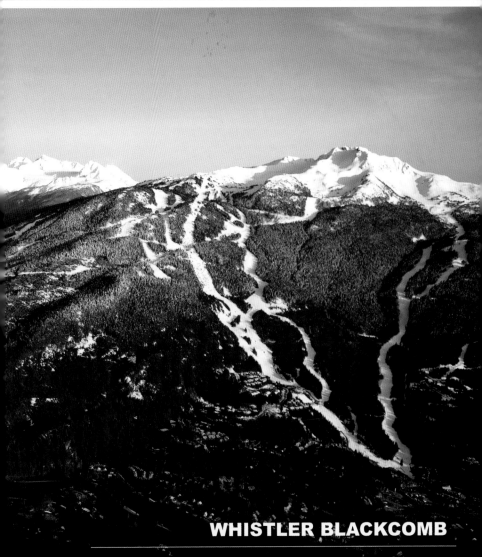

WHISTLER BLACKCOMB

An aerial view of the resort showing the staggering amount of alpine terrain available. Alta Lake is in the foreground, Whistler Creekside is on the far right, Whistler Village is on the left and the two ski areas, Blackcomb and Whistler, are shown from left to right, respectively.

About This Book

When the Ski and Snowboard Guide to Whistler Blackcomb came out in 2004, it was the first book of its kind in the ski industry. Despite our optimism, the naysayers were confused by the new concept, insisting that no one would buy the book when there was a perfectly good trail map available for free. Within months of release, however, the book caught fire, and local shops were frantically placing orders just to keep it on the shelves. Fast-forward seven years and the first edition has emerged as a Canadian bestseller. More than 20,000 people have disagreed with the naysayers!

So why have so many people found the book invaluable? Probably because Whistler and Blackcomb possess over 8,000 skiable acres, three glaciers, 12 alpine bowls and 34 lifts. These are two huge mountains, and finding your way around can be very confusing even with careful consultation of the trail map. Without someone showing you the goods, it can take the better part of a season just to figure out what your favorite runs are and how to access them. In short, anyone coming for a week-long vacation has to learn pretty fast. This book is an attempt to remedy this fact by presenting detailed information about the ski area in a usable format.

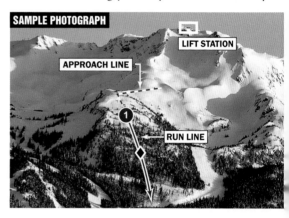

How To Use This Book

You have purchased the ultimate reference for skiers and snowboarders wishing to maximize their experience at Whistler Blackcomb. The book provides an overview of

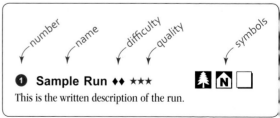

the advanced and expert terrain and is organized around specific chairlifts and zones. Run and access information is presented in a number of ways, including aerial photographs, symbols and text. The aerial photographs are superimposed with labels and markings and are an excellent tool for choosing what area you want to explore. The symbols provide a significant amount of information at a glance. Please refer to the symbol key to familiarize yourself with the definitions. The written text provides further information that photographs or symbols cannot.

Trail Designations

Many people find the blue runs at Whistler to be as hard as the black-diamond runs at other ski areas. So how do they classify the runs at Whistler Blackcomb? Trails receive a difficulty rating based on an evaluation of the slope's width, average gradient and the steepest 30 metres. A simple rating of green, blue or black does not do justice to the variety of terrain at Whistler Blackcomb, therefore, we have added double-black-diamond and triple-black-diamond ratings to this guide. Remember, with the increase in difficulty comes an increase in the risk of longer, more hazardous falls.

- ● Novice
- ■ Intermediate
- ◆ Advanced
- ◆◆ Expert
- ◆◆◆ Super expert

Quality Ratings

The runs in this book are given a quality rating, defined as follows:

★ Average run
★★ Very good run
★★★ Excellent run

This book is designed to work in conjunction with the mountain trail map or digital apps for smartphones. Trail maps are available free of charge throughout the resort and through your smartphone platform's marketplace.

Symbols

☐ Tick box

E Run aspect

▥ Regularly groomed

Good cruising

🌲 Tree skiing

Hike up

Jump in

Scary/exposed

☠ Very dangerous

Avalanche debris

Requires lots of snow

Cut bank hazard

Cliff hazard

Cornice hazard

Crevasse hazard

Traverse line hazard

Furthering Your Enjoyment of Whistler Blackcomb

Before heading up the hill for the day, make sure you check the snow report, either online or over the phone. The crucial numbers are as follows:

> Whistler Blackcomb Snowphone: (604) 932-4211 or (800) 766-0449, toll free
> Blackcomb Patrol Snow Report: (604) 935-5596

Calling the report will answer the following questions:

- ❏ How much new snow is there?
- ❏ What is the current and forecast weather on the hill?
- ❏ Is avalanche control being performed?
- ❏ What runs have been groomed?
- ❏ Are there any special events?

With this information in mind, you will be able to determine everything from which skis to use, what clothing to wear and which runs to ride first. If avalanche control is being conducted, there will likely be a delay in opening the upper mountain. Once you get on the hill, check out the light boards that are placed around the mountain. By checking the boards, you will find out which lifts are open, how long the lines are at each of the lifts and which lifts are on standby. As you know, on powder days timing is everything. You will want to anticipate which lifts are opening next in order to get your fair share of fresh snow. Here is the typical (yet certainly not guaranteed) order of lift openings after avalanche clearance.

Whistler: Roundhouse Zone and below—Harmony Express Chair—Peak Chair—Symphony Chair

Blackcomb: Wizard / Solar Coaster Chairs—Jersey Cream Express Chair—Crystal Chair—Seventh Heaven Express Chair—Glacier Express Chair—Showcase T-Bar

BlackDiamondEquipment.com

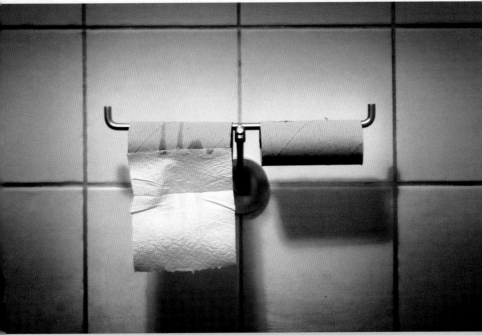

EVER BEEN **STUCK?**

NOW IMAGINE THAT, BUT FOR 45 MINUTES WITH NO AIR.

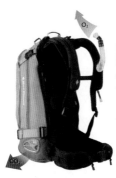

AVALUNG

The average avalanche rescue takes longer than your 15-minute air supply lasts.

By pulling air from the surrounding snowpack, the **AvaLung** allows you to breathe for nearly an hour, increasing your odds of survival.

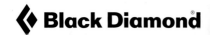

2010 Winter Olympics

If Whistler wasn't already on the map as an international ski destination, it officially arrived on the global scene in February, 2010. Vancouver may have been the official host city for the 2010 Winter Olympics, but the majority of the medals were earned in Whistler. The alpine skiing competitions were held on the Dave Murray Downhill and Franz's Run on Whistler Mountain, and the venues did not disappoint. Known as the glamour event of the Games, the women's downhill competition provided some spectacular crashes along with amazing and courageous performances by two American superstars, Lindsey Vonn (gold) and Julia Mancuso (silver), skiing the 2.9-km course on Franz's in the scorching times of 1:44:19 and 1:44:45, respectively. After the race, Canada's Emily Brydon tipped her hat to the long and difficult course by commenting, "The reason we are seeing so much carnage is just because we are so exhausted at the end."

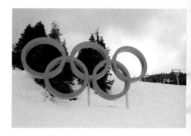

© KEVIN HODDER

On the men's side, Swiss dark horse Didier Défago shocked the world as he edged out the usual suspects, Norway's Aksel Lund Svindal (silver) and American bad boy Bode Miller (bronze). "I know this was a surprise to some people," said Défago, 32, the oldest winner of an Olympic downhill, "but not to me, I told my family I wanted to bring home a little more weight in my luggage. Just a little … like something gold!" The Dave Murray Downhill is the second-longest FIS downhill course in the world, dropping 870 m over 3.2 km. Racers complete the course with approximately 30 turns and can reach speeds of 140 km per hour. To put that in perspective, if you drove at that pace on the Sea to Sky Highway, you would be eligible for a $483 fine for excessive speeding!

Both of these racetracks are also blue-chip cruising runs when freshly groomed. Usually one or the other is rolled every night and can be a real treat to ride, especially with a few centimeters of fresh snow on top. In order to ski the men's course, simply access the Dave Murray Downhill from the top of the Garbanzo Express and follow it to the open area near tower nine of the Creekside Gondola. This area is known as the Timing Flats and was the finish line for all Olympic alpine events. The women's course is a bit trickier to navigate. It starts at the top of Wild Card and flows into Franz's Run above the intersection with Highway 86. The course then follows Franz's until it reaches a little cut away called Frandola, at which point it merges with the Dave Murray Downhill and arrives at the Timing Flats. The only real remnants of the Games still standing on the hill are the bright-green rings above the Timing Flats. It makes a popular photo spot.

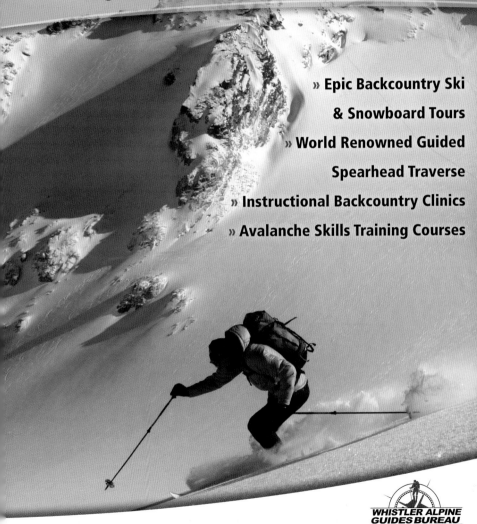

Avoiding Lineups

On powder days, you will most likely have to deal with a few lift lines if you want to put yourself in the fray for first tracks. On other days, there are some basic principles for avoiding lines on the hill. Many people prescribe the philosophy of "get up, stay up, eat smart". Since your biggest chance of getting tangled in a lift line is at the start of the day in the valley, it is crucial to get to the base early on weekends and holidays. You may also want to consider buying a ticket for Fresh Tracks Breakfast atop Whistler Mountain. For about $18, you can load the Gondola at 7:30, enjoy a buffet breakfast at the Roundhouse and hit the slopes before the rest of the skiers have arrived. Hey, why not let the queue form in the valley while you're shredding pow in the alpine.

Once on the upper mountain, stay up top until the morning rush is over. If you want to ride down to the village for lunch or take a ripper on Peak to Creek, make sure you check the light board before going too low. You could be heading into a major traffic jam if you descend too early. The "eat smart" component of the slogan has nothing to do with nutrition but a lot to do with timing. If you can make it part of your daily strategy to avoid the restaurants between the hours of noon and 2 o'clock you will probably be able skip any of the congestion. Whether you want to eat early or late, the choice is up to you, but make sure you are skiing instead of sitting in the middle of the day.

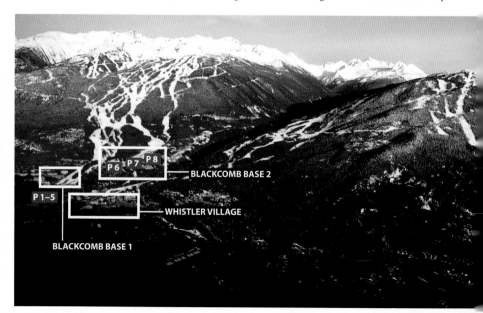

Parking

What was once a nonissue has become the first challenge of the day. And you thought those triple-black-diamond runs were tough!

The Creekside underground parking garage offers a convenient, covered and, at least for the time being, free option for motorists heading up to Whistler. The benefits beyond monetary can include a less lengthy exodus at the end of your day if you are heading south, since you completely avoid the Village. The downside is that the lift capacity is not fast enough to handle the potential volume of the lots. On busy days, this can result in lineups that stretch past the shops of Franz's Trail. One strategy is to pull into the lot and send a runner up to check the length of the line before committing to starting your day at Creekside.

Village Day Lots 1, 2, 3, 4 and 5 were once the bread-and-butter parking option for all skiers. After the 2010 Olympic Games, however, the lots became pay parking with rates of $8.00 per day. All five lots require payment, despite protests by the people of Whistler during the summer of 2011.

There are three more parking lots at Base 2 on Blackcomb. Lot 6 is at the midstation of the Excalibur Gondola, Lot 7 is above the staff-housing complex past the valley main-

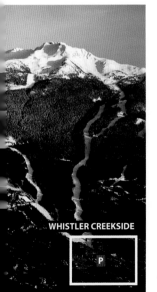

WHISTLER CREEKSIDE

tenance shop, and Lot 8 is adjacent to the Whistler Sliding Centre and Tube Park. All three are free and offer skiing directly to and from the lot, requiring minimal walking in ski boots. These are now the most sought-after spots in the Valley and have changed the traffic flow of where people park and upload. If you choose to park here, your best bet for faster access up the hill and smaller lift lines is to ski down to the Wizard Express rather than load the Excalibur at midstation or the Village Gondola to Whistler.

Since it appears that pay parking is here to stay, it looks like the early birds will continue to catch those precious free spots at Creekside and Base 2. Lets just hope Whistler Blackcomb will remain sensible and avoid going the route of the municipality's money-grab parking scheme.

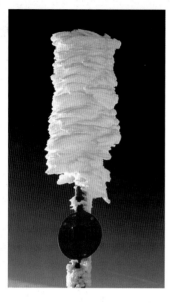

On Hill Signage

Most signs are self-explanatory. The following, however, is the interpretation and consequences of the signage at Whistler Blackcomb.

Ski Area Boundary—This sign indicates the border of Whistler Blackcomb's patrolled area. Skiing or riding outside the area is done at your own risk. It is your responsibility to have the adequate knowledge to travel safely in avalanche terrain and to carry the essential rescue gear. People who require evacuation from the backcountry will be charged for their rescue.

Early/Late Season Boundary—Temporary "Area Boundary" signs are posted within the ski area during early and late portions of the season. These boundaries denote parts of the hill that do not have sufficient snow and feature extensive hazards. As a result, there are no hazard markings, no patrols, and no sweep of these areas at the end of the day. As the snow coverage permits these boundaries disappear.

Permanently Closed—Permanent closure signs at Whistler Blackcomb indicate areas of the mountain that are NEVER open. These are areas within the ski area that are determined to be unsuitable for skiing. The danger of entering these areas often extends beyond the risk to the offending skier or rider, because their actions threaten skiers on runs below. Passes will be revoked from anyone who disobeys these signs.

Closed/Avalanche Hazard—These signs are used to temporarily close areas within the ski area. Avalanche closures keep guests out of harm's way during active avalanche control (explosives!) or when the hazard grows too high and control is not possible. Passes will be revoked from anyone who disobeys these signs.

Closed—Runs are closed for several reasons. These reasons may include: thin snow cover, ditches or holes, fallen trees, races or other events are taking place, terrain parks are not yet ready to open, snow making or other machinery is operating, etc. Passes will be revoked from anyone who disobeys these signs.

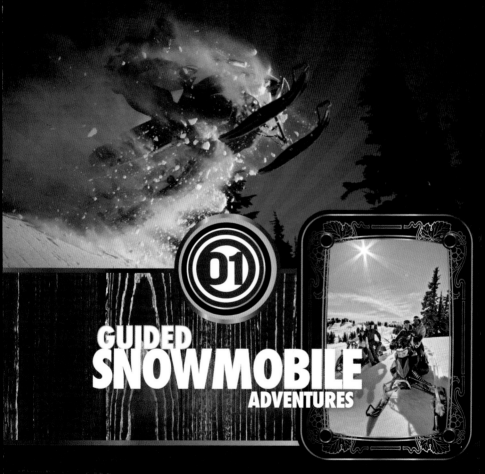

CANADIAN01.COM

BLACKCOMB MTN I CALLAGHAN BACKCOUNTRY

CANADIAN

SNOWMOBILE I DOGSLED I SNOWSHOE I FONDUE

01

GUIDED
SNOWMOBILE
ADVENTURES

WHISTLER B.C.

604.938.1616

FRONT DESK: IN THE CARLETON LODGE BESIDE THE LONGHORN

Code of Conduct

Lets face it: powder snow is a perishable and addictive substance, and like all things in those categories, a frenzied state can arise from its pursuit. In the past, we have witnessed a few isolated incidents of yelling and pushing between crazed powder fiends. All of these situations are preventable if a basic code of ethics is allowed to prevail.

Lift lines—Everyone will get to the top eventually. This isn't Europe, so don't push, shove, butt in or let your friends in. Besides, everyone knows there are no friends on powder days!

Choosing your line—If you're still refining your powder-riding skills, choose a moderate slope that matches your ability. In new-snow conditions, leave the classic steep lines for those who can shred them with fluid proficiency. Don't worry; you'll be there soon enough!

Bootpacks—A bootpack is a place where people walk uphill in order to access areas not directly serviced by the lifts. An example is Spanky's Ladder at the top of the Glacier Ex-

Safety

Know the alpine responsibility code. You will be held accountable to it! In addition, it is advisable to:

- ❏ Avoid skiing or riding alone in expert terrain, especially in the trees!

- ❏ Know where you are at all times! If in doubt, ask the ski patrol! Each year, many passes are revoked, and many injuries occur because people unwittingly enter closed runs or terrain beyond their abilities.

- ❏ Respect the Slow Zones as posted on both mountains. These are the areas frequented by families and those new to the sport. Remember, you were there once, too!

- ❏ Slow down and ride with extra caution when the visibility is poor or the snow surface is hard. Collisions are shockingly common!

- ❏ Protect yourself from sunburn and frostbite. The effect of ultraviolet radiation and cold temperatures can be magnified in the mountains.

- ❏ Wear a helmet. Although they have limitations, they could save your life!

press chair. These areas can become quite congested on powder days. If you become too tired to keep walking up the bootpack, step off to the side while you rest and let the people behind you pass.

Ride your own line—Be conscious of not diverting from your chosen line into someone else's. A 20-centimetre powder day is no time to be zigzagging across the slope in search of better snow. Make your choice at the top!

"Locals"—Just because you moved here from Ontario last July doesn't mean you have more right to a certain area than someone who is here on vacation. Hey, you choose to live in a resort that receives 2 million skier visits per season. There are going to be lots of other skiers on the hill, and most of them deserve your respect.

T-Bars—If you aren't familiar with riding T-bars, a powder day is not the time to learn! Ask the lift attendant for instructions at a quieter time.

Smoking—There is no smoking allowed in the restaurants, patios or lift lines at Whistler Blackcomb. Inhale that clean mountain air instead!

Respect the snow, the mountain and the other riders!

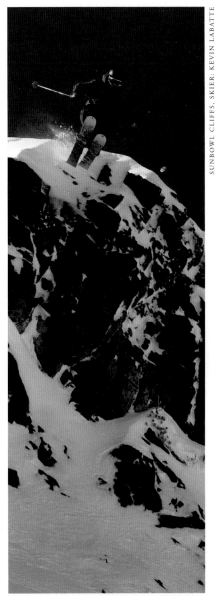

SUNBOWL CLIFFS, SKIER: KEVIN LABATTE

ARMCHAIR BOOKS

4205 Village Square ~ 604-932-5557 ~ armchair@whistlerbooks.com

Armchair Books is a family run bookstore located in the heart of Whistler Village.

We offer a full range of:

- Magazines
- Kids books
- Maps
- Guide books
- Cook Books
- Fiction
- History
- Biography
- Stationary
- And fabulous titles like Malcolm Gladwell's...

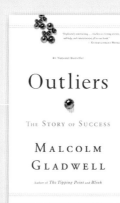

Malcolm Gladwell
Collected Box Set:

ISBN 9780316123099

$85.00

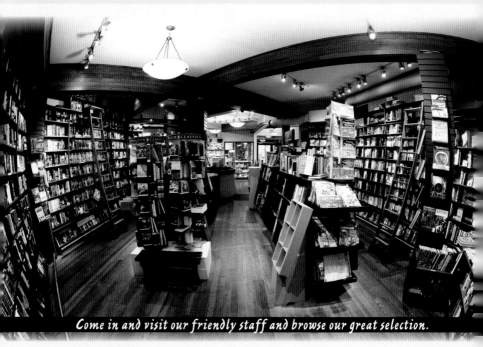

Come in and visit our friendly staff and browse our great selection.

Avalanche Control

The avalanche control program is designed to reduce the hazard within the ski area by intentionally starting avalanches before the skiing public is present. The individual in charge of directing the program is the Avalanche Forecaster. The Forecaster will begin by assessing the snow stability and avalanche hazard through a detailed analysis of several factors including snowfall amounts, temperature, winds, humidity and weather forecasts. The Forecaster will then direct a crew of ski patrollers to control the hazard in an efficient manner so that the terrain is open as soon as possible. This crew will leave the valley before dawn and will be skiing before the majority of us have had our second cup of coffee.

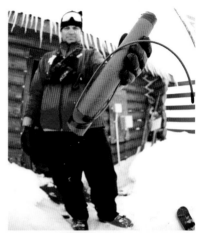

Most avalanche control involves the use of explosives to initiate the activity. It is not uncommon for 200 kg of explosives to be used on the mountains during a morning when the avalanche hazard is high.

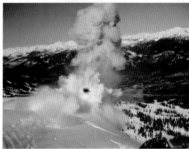

The patrollers, working in teams of two, are assigned specific "routes" which they are responsible for controlling. They will deposit their explosives on the slopes using several methods of deployment. The primary method is called a "hand charge". A hand charge is simply a stick of explosive with a fuse and igniter cap. The teams literally ski along the ridge tops with a pack full of explosives. When they arrive at the point above a predetermined target they light the fuse and throw the hand charge onto the slope or

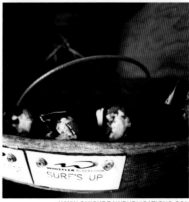

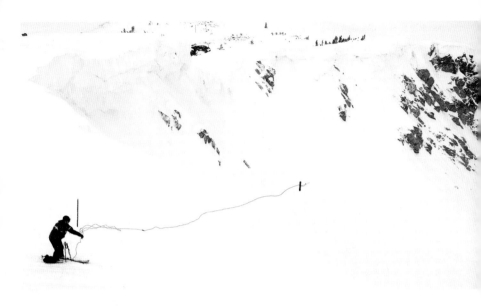

cornice. Once the fuse is lit the team has two and a half minutes to get to a safe spot, plug their ears and wait.

If the terrain is too difficult (or dangerous) to access on skis, then an aerial "bomb-tram" may be utilized. A bomb-tram is a permanent structure that is installed across a span of terrain and works like a giant clothesline. After explosives are attached to the line and the fuse is lit, the patroller can "wheel" the assembly out over the desired place on the slope. Bomb-trams are visible in the alpine areas of both mountains. The most visible tram is off to your left as you ride the Peak Chair past tower 10.

"Avalaunchers" are permanently installed guns that are used to shoot explosive project-iles at otherwise inaccessible pieces of terrain. An avalauncher is operated by releasing a measured amount of pressurized nitrogen gas through a barrel thus propelling a pro-jectile toward a target like a giant peashooter. This peashooter, however, can lob a one-kilogram rocket over a distance of 2,000 metres! There are currently seven avalaunchers installed at Whistler Blackcomb.

When the weather permits, the most effective and time-efficient method of delivering explosives to the slopes is by dropping them out of a helicopter. "Helibombing" involves three patrollers in the helicopter: the Bombardier, the Explosives Prep and the Recorder. A fourth patroller remains on the ground assembling the explosives for each round.

The most utilized non-explosive method of avalanche control is "ski-cutting". This method involves skiing across the start zones of avalanche paths to initiate activity. This can be a very dangerous technique and is most often used by the patrol to remove small "pocket' avalanches that were not initiated by earlier explosive control.

It is easy to perceive avalanche control as a "dream job" however it can be an intense experience. Imagine an hour within a helicopter, hovering close to the ground with the door open and the smoke of burning fuses filling the cabin. Add a little turbulence from winds and you have the perfect recipe for motion sickness! The next morning you may be expected to ski double-black diamond terrain in the dark with a pack full of bombs. Needless to say falling is not an option!

The avalanche control program is performed by a dedicated group of professionals with the mandate of opening the terrain as soon as possible. Please respect them for working hard behind the scenes and allowing us to access the goods!

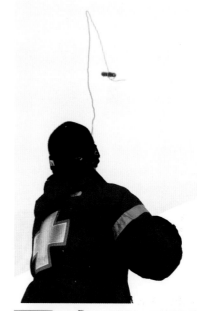

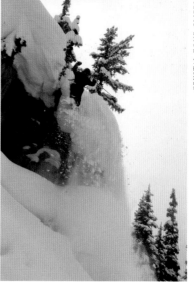

CRYSTAL ZONE CLIFFS

Hazards

Tree Wells—More people are killed in coastal snow regions by tree wells than by avalanches! A tree well is a phenomenon unique to big mountains with deep snow packs. A tree well forms when snow falling on evergreens accumulates between the trees but not around the tree trunk. As the snow is shed from the branches above it falls away from the tree creating a moat around the base of the tree. As the snow gets deeper so does the tree well.

The danger of the tree well exists when a person falls over in the snow and ends up with their body upside down in the tree well. As the person struggles to get out, the hole fills with snow, potentially burying the victim. Many people have died of suffocation in the wells of both large trees and small saplings. Unlike avalanches, tree wells cannot be reasonably controlled and the hazard exists anywhere on the mountain once the snow pack exceeds one metre (about three feet) in depth. When riding in the trees it is very important to maintain constant audible contact with everyone in your party. It is recommended that avid tree skiers have a whistle on their jackets for this purpose.

Cornices—These are formed when wind-transported snow is deposited on the lee aspect of a ridge. The dense snow forms meringue-like tongues that overhang the slopes below. Although the snow appears capable of supporting a skier's weight, it can fracture and drop the rider (and massive amounts of snow) over the edge and down the slope.

Entry into slopes guarded by cornices is tricky and dangerous business. Many of the runs described in this book involve negotiating an entry around a cornice. Whistler Blackcomb's avalanche control program includes the "trimming" of cornices with explosives. This preventative measure ensures that the cornices don't grow too big, but does not guarantee that they are safe to walk on or won't fall naturally with changing temperatures.

All cornices should be treated with respect and considered time bombs ready to collapse. The best way to gain access to the slope below a cornice is to stay well back from the edge and scout for any obvious entry that cuts in at a natural notch. If no such entry exists, it may be best to leave that line for another day.

Once the cornice has fallen onto the slope it poses a different kind of hazard. Cornice debris can range cubes the size of cinderblocks to Chevy truck-sized behemoths. When the light is flat or visibility is obscured by falling snow or fog, colliding with these solid chunks can be a real possibility. Be aware of this hazard and ski accordingly!

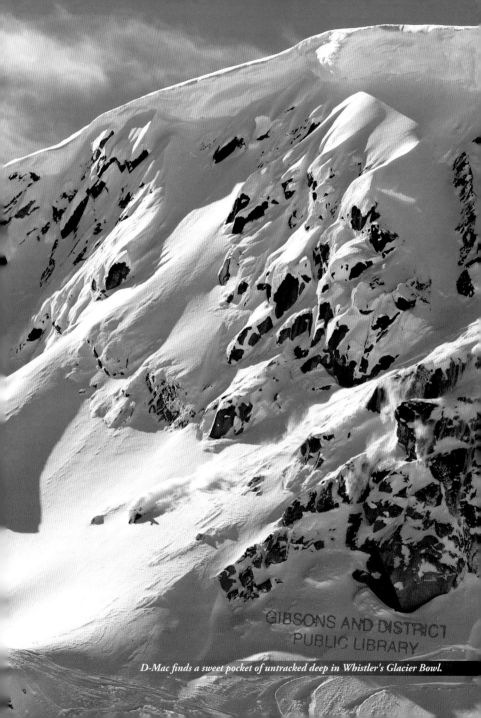

D-Mac finds a sweet pocket of untracked deep in Whistler's Glacier Bowl.

Backcountry Access

Whistler has developed a reputation for being one of the best locations in North America for lift-accessed backcountry skiing. Areas such as Cowboy Ridge, Fissile, Husume, Corona, the Poop Chutes, Disease Ridge and DOA have become popular destinations for skiers seeking the next level of adventure from their on-mountain experience. Of course, anyone proceeding beyond the ski area boundary is doing so completely at his or her own risk, and if you are in doubt as to whether a run is within the ski area boundary or not, it is your responsibility to ask the ski patrol. The backcountry is an unpatrolled space, and no avalanche control has been performed to reduce the hazard. It is important that anyone leaving the ski area has the experience, education and equipment required to mitigate personal risk. If you are not highly experienced at backcountry travel and rescue, it is recommended that you hire a certified guide to negotiate the hazards for you. Guides can be hired at the Whistler Alpine Guides Bureau (Whistlerguides.com) in the village. The bureau also holds regular avalanche-skills training and wilderness first-aid courses that are highly recommended.

The ski patrol posts a very well written avalanche advisory under the Weather and Cams tab at Whistlerblackcomb.com. This page also links to the Canadian Avalanche Centre bulletin for the region. Both are required reading for anyone choosing to travel in the Whistler backcountry.

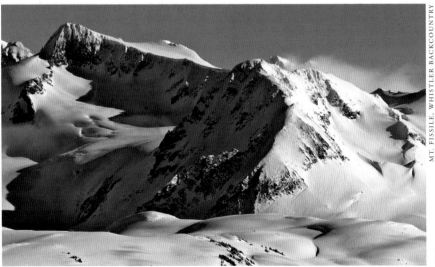

MT. FISSILE, WHISTLER BACKCOUNTRY

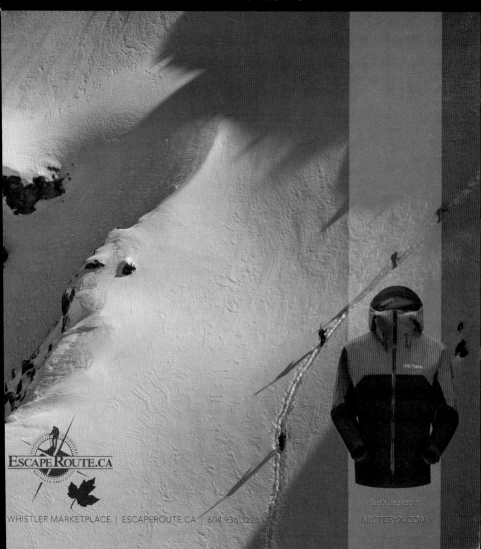

Weather

The weather in Whistler is a direct result of the region's unique geography and winter's typical atmospheric conditions.

The coast of British Columbia stretches for almost 800 kilometres and is dominated by the rugged spine of the Coast Mountains. Directly to the west of these mountains lies the largest body of water on the planet, the Pacific Ocean—a constant source of heat and moisture.

In winter, the circulation of atmospheric winds offshore of B.C. results from two semi-permanent features: the Pacific High, which is usually centralized between Hawaii and California, and the Aleutian Low in the Gulf of Alaska (Figure 1). The clockwise circulation of the Pacific High and the counterclockwise rotation of the Aleutian Low lead to a predominantly western flow of weather onto the coast of the province. This moist, warm westerly flow slams into the Coast Mountains and is forced upward and cools. As the air cools, its capacity to retain moisture drops and precipitation results.

Figure 1 *Map of North America showing typical positions of the Aleutian Low and Pacific High during the winter months. The red arrows show wind direction and the grey lines are surface pressure.*

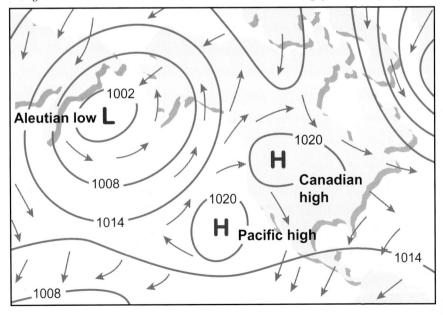

Of course, this being nature, anomalies exist within the predominant pattern. The Arctic Outflow and the Pineapple Express are examples of conditions that usually occur every winter but are not prevalent. An Arctic Outflow environment occurs when a powerful and frigid anticyclone establishes over the province's interior. In Whistler, an outflow produces dry,

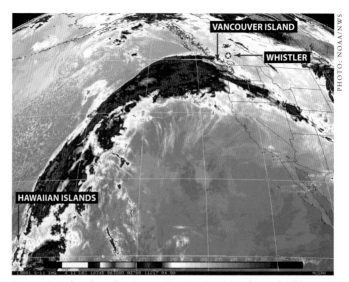

VANCOUVER ISLAND

WHISTLER

HAWAIIAN ISLANDS

PHOTO: NOAA/NWS

Figure 2 *Infrared satellite image showing the classic form of a Pineapple Express. To Whistler, from Hawaii with love!*

clear and cold conditions, which sometimes follow an intense "power flurry" of snow. An easterly flow will generally result and winds can be high in the alpine, creating a serious risk of frostbite to skiers.

On the other end of the spectrum lies the dreaded Pineapple Express (Figure 2), which brings warm temperatures and intense precipitation to the region. As the name would imply, these systems originate near the Hawaiian Islands and, in some cases, they can stall over the region, serving the worst conditions Whistler has to offer—slashing rain into the alpine! Eccentric locals swear they can smell coconuts during these conditions.

A good place to get a summary of the alpine weather forecast is the weather tab at Whistlerblackcomb.com. This site will outline the current and forecasted conditions along with an estimate of how much snow will accumulate throughout the next five days. Conspiracy theorists can rest assured that Environment Canada, as opposed to the Whistler Blackcomb marketing department, provides this forecast. Other good sources of weather and climate information are Whistlerpeak.com, Whistlerweather. org and Weatheroffice.gc.ca.

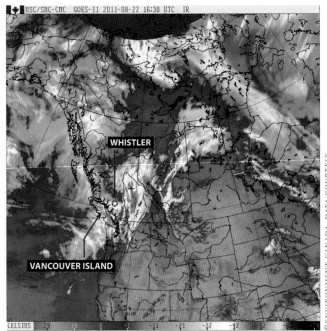

MSC/SMC-CMC GOES-11 2011-08-22 16:30 UTC   IR

WHISTLER

VANCOUVER ISLAND

CELSIUS

©ENVIRONMENT CANADA, DATA COURTESY OF NOAA, 2011

Figure 3 *Infrared satellite image showing an example of weather activity over the western part of Canada. Vancouver Island and Whistler are marked for reference.*

Another great way to stay abreast of weather that is approaching the coast of British Columbia is to routinely review satellite images that are available online. The picture of principal concern for Whistler skiers comes from the Geostationary Operational Environmental Satellite that is positioned over the western section of the continent at an elevation of over 35,000 kilometres. Known as GOES-West, this satellite performs a geosynchronous orbit over the Earth. In lay terms, this means that it observes the planet from the same place at all times and provides half-hourly reports of the environment from this perspective. Serious weather freaks are fanatical about checking the images that GOES-West provides.

If you want to look for yourself, review the GOES-West Western Canada IR satellite image at Weatheroffice.gc.ca (Figure 3). It's updated hourly and shows the weather that is either imminently approaching the coast of British Columbia or has already landed. Enlarge this image (by clicking on it) to get a close-up of the region. You can roughly locate the Whistler area on the image by visually drawing a horizontal line

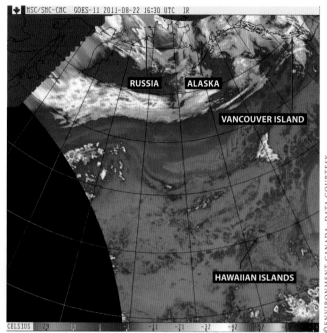

MSC/SMC-CMC   GOES-11 2011-08-22 16:30 UTC   IR

RUSSIA   ALASKA

VANCOUVER ISLAND

HAWAIIAN ISLANDS

CELSIUS   29   19   8   -1   -11   -21   -32   -42   -52

©ENVIRONMENT CANADA. DATA COURTESY OF NOAA, 2011

Figure 4 *Infrared satellite image showing an example of weather activity over the North Pacific. This helps provide information about upcoming weather activity along the British Columbia coastline.*

from the centre of Vancouver Island east into the province. Whistler lies on this line approximately 100 kilometres from the Straight of Georgia, the channel that separates Vancouver Island from the mainland.

As well, check out the GOES-West North Pacific IR satellite image (Figure 4) at the same website. This image, also updated hourly, presents a view of the weather that is approaching from far out over the Pacific. Look at the bar at the bottom of the image, which details what temperatures the colors represent. Remember, the lower the infrared temperature, the more moisture there is in the atmosphere. The more moisture there is in the atmosphere, the more moisture is available to fall as precipitation onshore.

Finally, look at the 24-hour compilation of infrared images from GOES-West called the West CONUS Loop at Goes.noaa.gov. This loop is a very useful tool for predicting how the systems over the Pacific are tracking and where the majority of the precipitation will fall. Sometimes, you can see that the storms are probably going to track just south of Whistler, while other times, you can tell that we are right in the line of fire. Have a look at the date-and-time bar atop the image so that you know what times the loop represents. The time is stated in Greenwich Mean Time, so you will have to subtract eight hours (seven hours once daylight saving time has begun) to equal Pacific Standard Time.

Although the knowledge gained from learning how to interpret the various satellite images is invaluable, some simpler rules of thumb apply and provide a quick prediction of conditions in Whistler from afar. For instance, if the temperature in Vancouver is 7° C or colder and it is raining, expect snowfall in Whistler Village, but if the temperature in Vancouver is closer to 10° C, freezing temperatures at the top of the Wizard Express on Blackcomb are more likely. Use the adjacent temperature and snowfall charts to help get a feel for how the mountain conditions change throughout the winter months.

VALLEY TEMPERATURE AVERAGES

Month	High	Low	High	Low
December	-1°C	-5°C	30°F	23°F
January	-2°C	-8°C	28°F	18°F
February	3°C	-5°C	37°F	23°F
March	8°C	-3°C	46°F	27°F
April	11°C	-2°C	52°F	36°F
May	17°C	7°C	62°F	44°F

ALPINE TEMPERATURE AVERAGES

Month	High	Low	High	Low
December	-5°C	-9°C	23°F	16°F
January	-5°C	-10°C	23°F	14°F
February	-3°C	-7°C	27°F	19°F
March	-1°C	-5°C	30°F	23°F
April	1°C	-4°C	34°F	25°F
May	4°C	0°C	39°F	32°F

SNOWFALL AVERAGES

November	88 cm	35 in
December	284 cm	112 in
January	183 cm	72 in
February	109 cm	43 in
March	198 cm	78 in
April	118 cm	46 in
May	53 cm	21 in

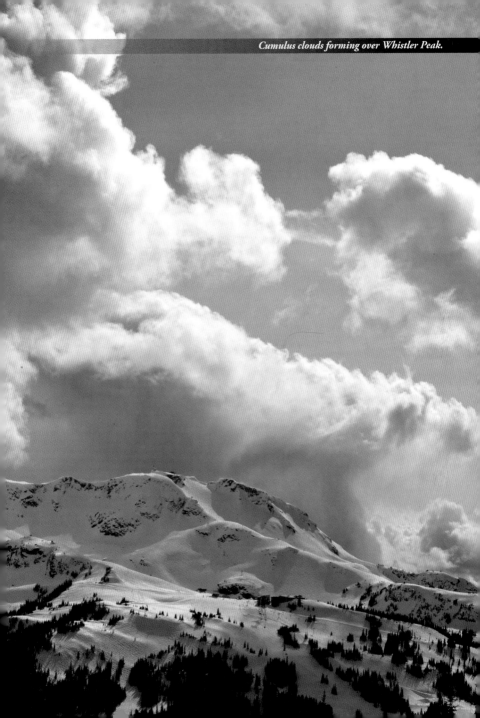
Cumulus clouds forming over Whistler Peak.

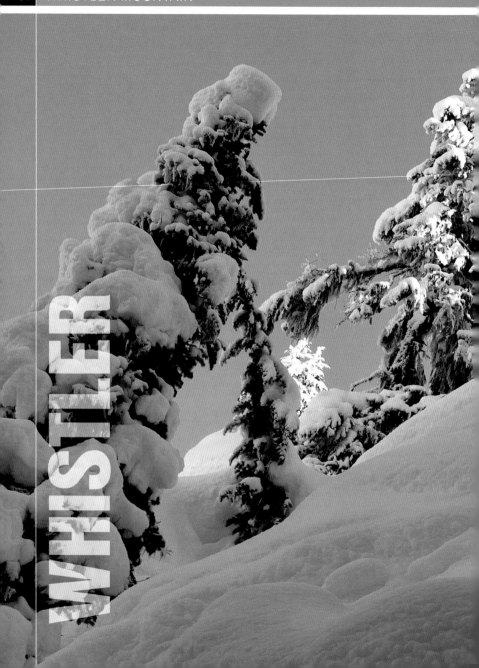

WHISTLER

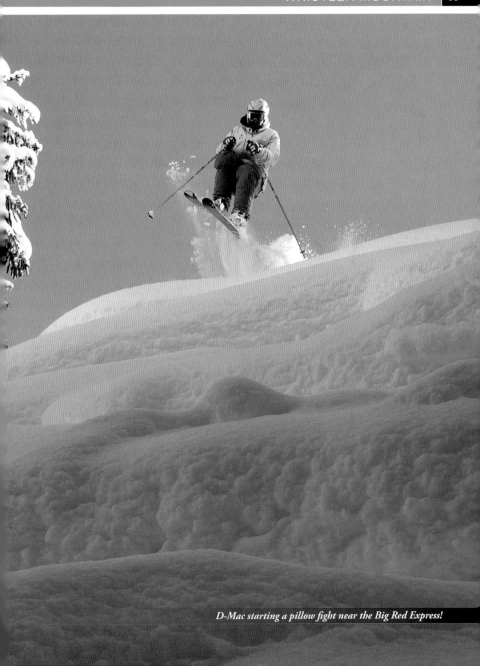

D-Mac starting a pillow fight near the Big Red Express!

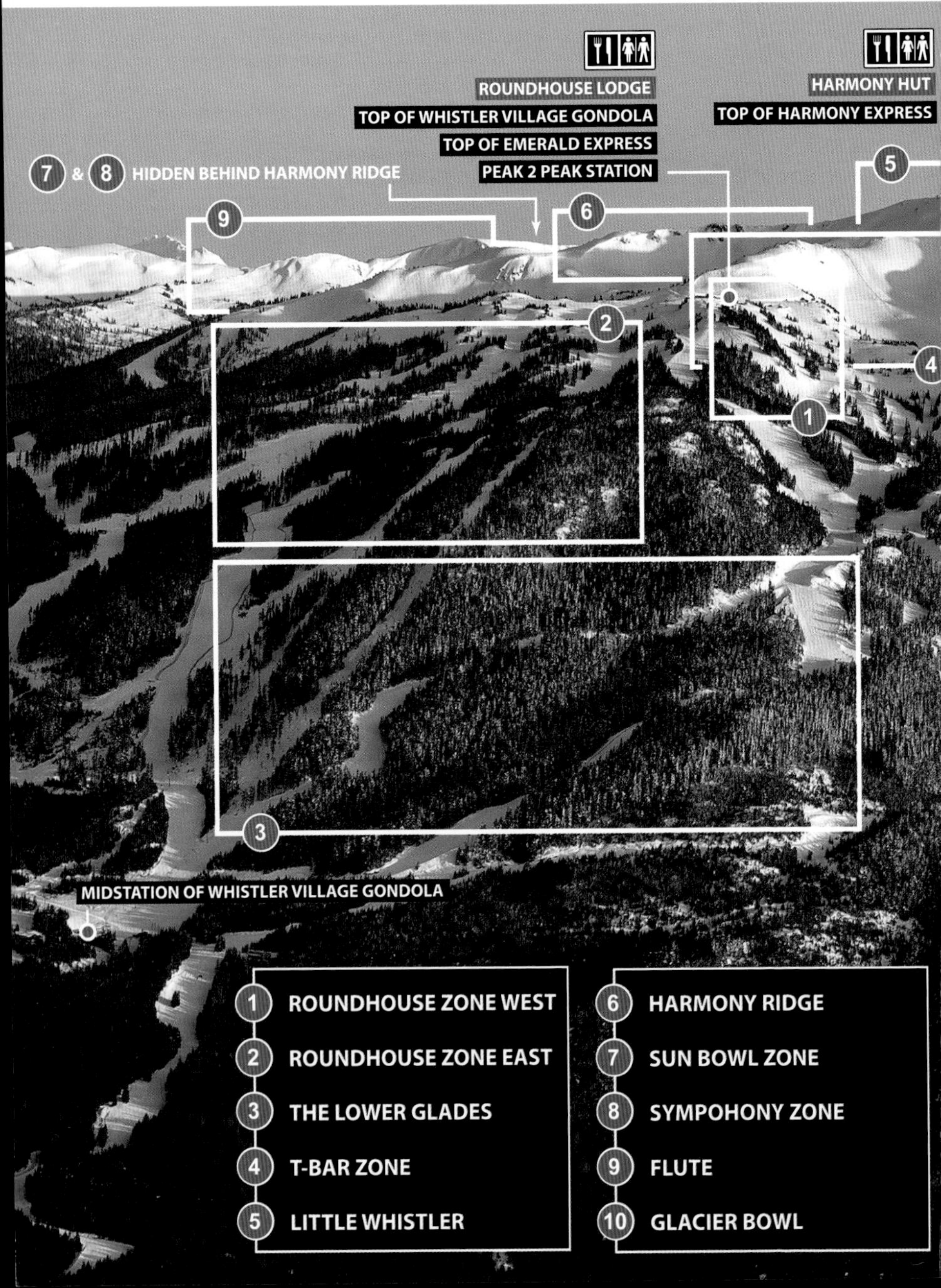

ROUNDHOUSE LODGE
TOP OF WHISTLER VILLAGE GONDOLA
TOP OF EMERALD EXPRESS
PEAK 2 PEAK STATION

HARMONY HUT
TOP OF HARMONY EXPRESS

7 & 8 HIDDEN BEHIND HARMONY RIDGE

9

5

6

2

4

1

3

MIDSTATION OF WHISTLER VILLAGE GONDOLA

1	ROUNDHOUSE ZONE WEST	6	HARMONY RIDGE
2	ROUNDHOUSE ZONE EAST	7	SUN BOWL ZONE
3	THE LOWER GLADES	8	SYMPOHONY ZONE
4	T-BAR ZONE	9	FLUTE
5	LITTLE WHISTLER	10	GLACIER BOWL

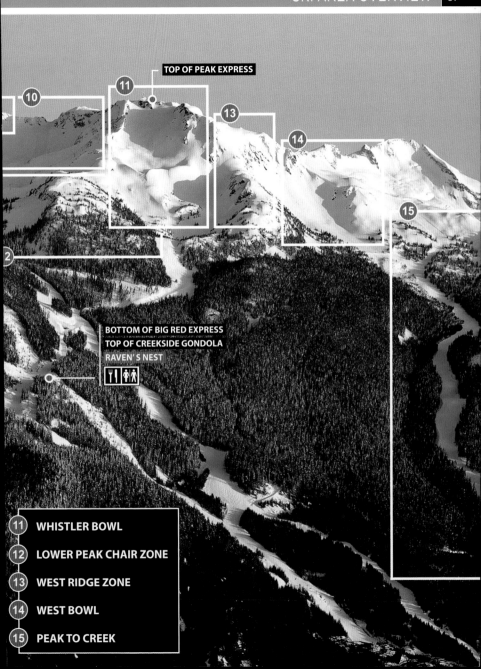

TOP OF PEAK EXPRESS

10

11

13

14

15

2

BOTTOM OF BIG RED EXPRESS
TOP OF CREEKSIDE GONDOLA
RAVEN'S NEST

11 WHISTLER BOWL

12 LOWER PEAK CHAIR ZONE

13 WEST RIDGE ZONE

14 WEST BOWL

15 PEAK TO CREEK

① Roundhouse Zone West

The Roundhouse Lodge is located at the top of the Whistler Village Gondola and adjacent to the tops of both the Emerald Express and Big Red Express chairs. The zone below the lodge, although dominated by intermediate and novice terrain, does contain some interesting runs. The beauty of the Roundhouse Zone is that it remains open in extremely inclement weather, which, let's face it, Whistler has its share of. If the T-Bars, Harmony Express and Peak Chair are closed because of weather, these runs may be your best option.

❶ Franz's Meadow ♦ ★★

A beautiful open bowl; deservedly popular! To get there from the Roundhouse, head down Pony Trail until it flattens out under the Big Red Express. From here, keep your elevation and traverse over to the meadow.

❷ Lower V.D. Chutes via the Goat Path ♦♦

Caution—There are a lot of ugly cliffs in the area below the Goat Path. Go with someone who knows the area until you have it figured out for yourself! The Goat Path can also be taken all the way over to the last pitch of Grande Finale, though it provides a short run after a long traverse.

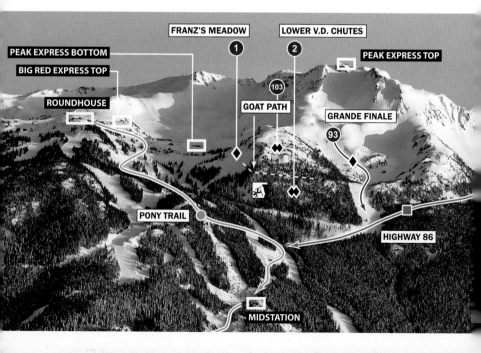

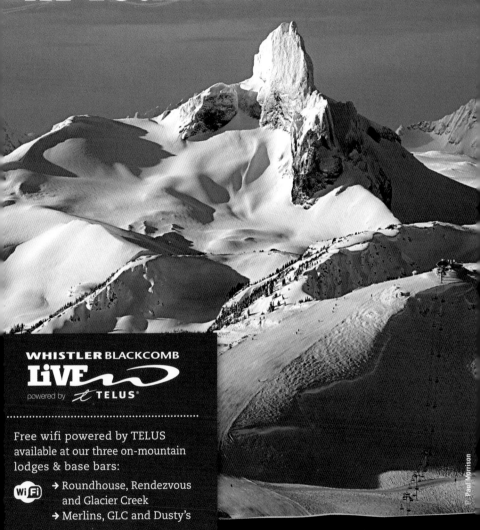

THE MOUNTAINS
AT YOUR FINGERTIPS

WHISTLER BLACKCOMB
LiVE
powered by *TELUS*®

Free wifi powered by TELUS
available at our three on-mountain
lodges & base bars:

Wi Fi
→ Roundhouse, Rendezvous
  and Glacier Creek
→ Merlins, GLC and Dusty's

DOWNLOAD OUR FREE APP NOW
whistlerblackcomb.com/app

P: Paul Morrison

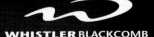

WHISTLER BLACKCOMB

❸ C.C. ♦ ★

Start from behind the top of the Whistler Village Gondola.

❹ Paleface ♦ ★

As for C.C.

❺ Wildcard ♦ ★

Made famous during the Vancouver 2010 Winter Olympics as the start of the women's downhill. It's a good run that links to Franz's.

❻ Jimmy's Joker ♦ ★

Access via Bear Cub. This run gets pretty bumped up, but it's fun with new snow. Like Wildcard, it drops you off on Franz's.

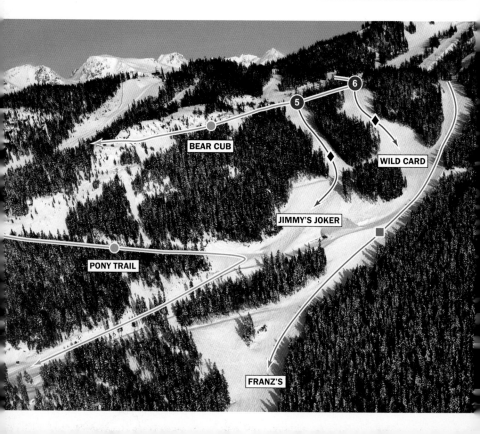

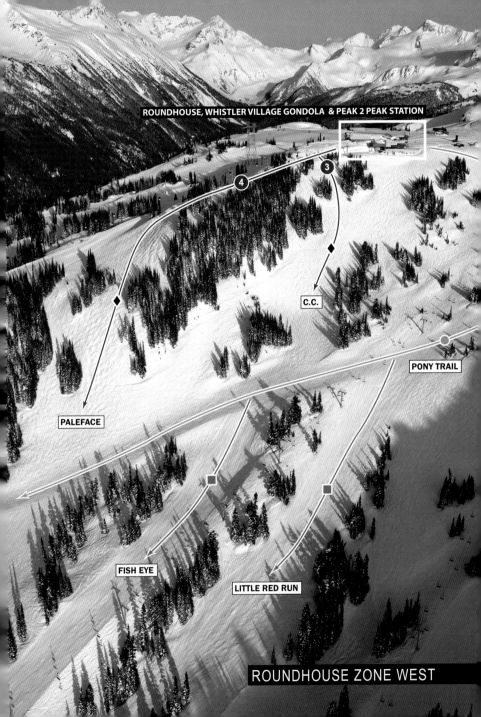

ROUNDHOUSE, WHISTLER VILLAGE GONDOLA & PEAK 2 PEAK STATION

4

3

C.C.

PONY TRAIL

PALEFACE

FISH EYE

LITTLE RED RUN

ROUNDHOUSE ZONE WEST

7 Goat's Gully ♦ ★

Once upon a time this was the Orange Chair lift line and it had all the qualities of a great mogul run: fall-line terrain, steep gradient near the top and a chair lift providing a consistent stream of spectators! She may not be in her heyday anymore, but this old goat can still kick back!

8 Insanity ♦♦ ★★

Insanity is technically a lift line only and not an official "ski run". According to the Whistler Blackcomb Safety Department, this means it may or may not have tower pads, trail markings or a sweep at the end of the day. Skiers and boarders have to accept a higher level of risk but will not have their passes removed for riding this run as long as it isn't marked at the top with a closed sign. Regardless of the confusing status, Insanity is a fun, varied ramble littered with well-spaced trees, cliffs and rocks. The upper section of this line starts at the point where the Big Red Express crosses Pony Trail and leads down to base of the lift. The lower and steeper section starts near the top of the Creekside Gondola and deposits skiers onto the Dave Murray Downhill. In the old days, skiing this terrain may have seemed "insane" to many but as time moves on, so changes the definition of what is "skiable". The upper section is a great ride on a powder day when you're waiting for the upper lifts to open.

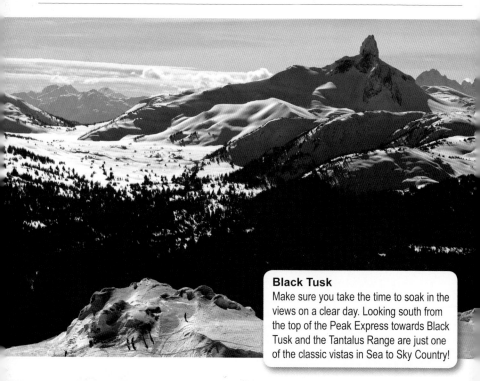

Black Tusk
Make sure you take the time to soak in the views on a clear day. Looking south from the top of the Peak Express towards Black Tusk and the Tantalus Range are just one of the classic vistas in Sea to Sky Country!

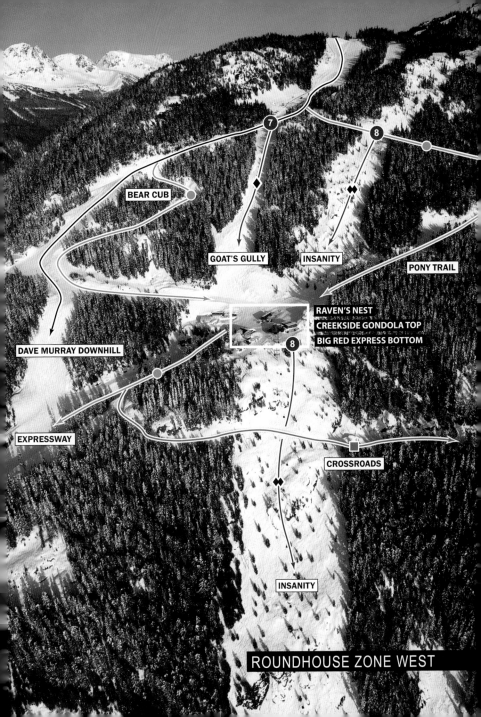

BEAR CUB

7

8

GOAT'S GULLY

INSANITY

PONY TRAIL

RAVEN'S NEST
CREEKSIDE GONDOLA TOP
BIG RED EXPRESS BOTTOM

8

DAVE MURRAY DOWNHILL

EXPRESSWAY

CROSSROADS

INSANITY

ROUNDHOUSE ZONE WEST

② Roundhouse Zone East

❾ Zudrell's ♦ ★

This is the Peak 2 Peak lift line between tower two and Sidewinder. It is named after Mathias Zudrell, a Doppelmayr engineer who was the first person to ride across the newly constructed gondola line between the two mountains.

❿ Ratfink ♦ ★

Some interesting steep rolls and cliffs.

⓫ Chunky's Choice ♦ ★

Considered a classic when bump skiing was the rage! Dust off that "daffy" with which you used to impress the chicks. Scott boots, Spalding skis and Schneider stretch pants required!

⓬ Dapper's Delight ♦ ★

The former Blue Chair lift line. A straight fall line shot with a good pitch.

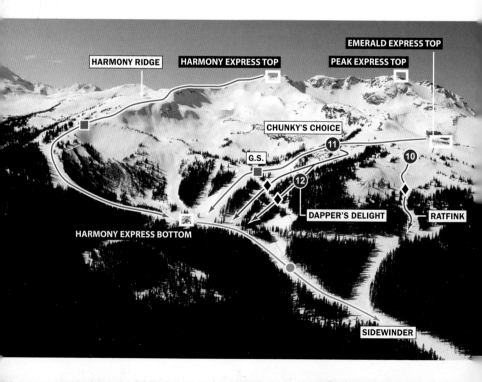

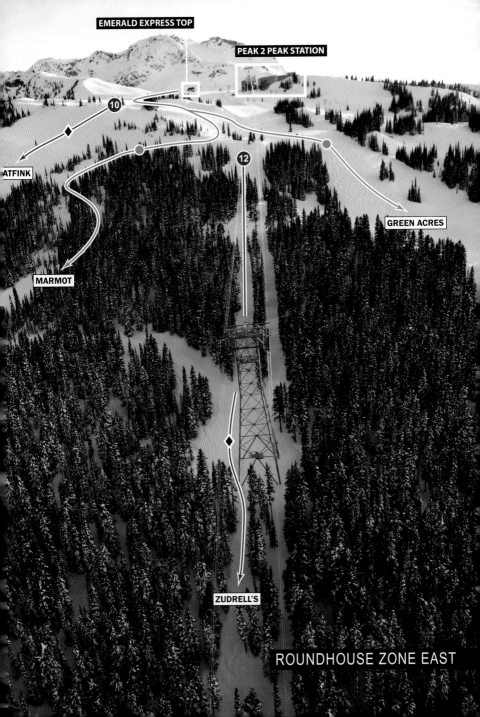

⑬ Seppo's ♦ ★

A ridiculously off fall line run that was named after one of the area's iconic residents, Seppo Makinen. It's a great option during a storm. Access Seppo's via the Garbanzo Express and look for the signs at the top.

⑭ Whistler Village Gondola Lift Line ♦ ★

As is the case with Insanity, this is technically a lift line only and not a designated "ski run". The patrol may or may not place pads on the towers or markings on the hazards and may not give it a sweep at the end of the day. You have to look out for yourself a bit more but as long as there isn't a closed sign at the top, you won't have your pass yanked for skiing it. In the right conditions and with ample coverage, this is a nice long run that often receives fewer tracks than others in the zone.

⑮ Garbanzo Lift Line ♦ ★

This is a long fall line shot with undulating terrain and a few cliffs thrown in for good measure. This lift line can be a riot with new snow. The line ends abruptly at a point where you have to sneak through the trees to Bear Paw (it was designed as a lift line not a ski run, after all). It's kind of like the movie No Country for Old Men: Ninety-five percent of it's great, but the ending sucks!

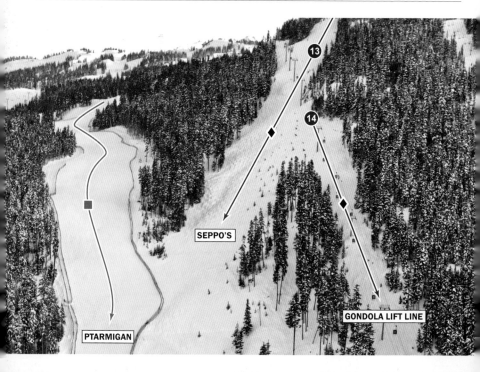

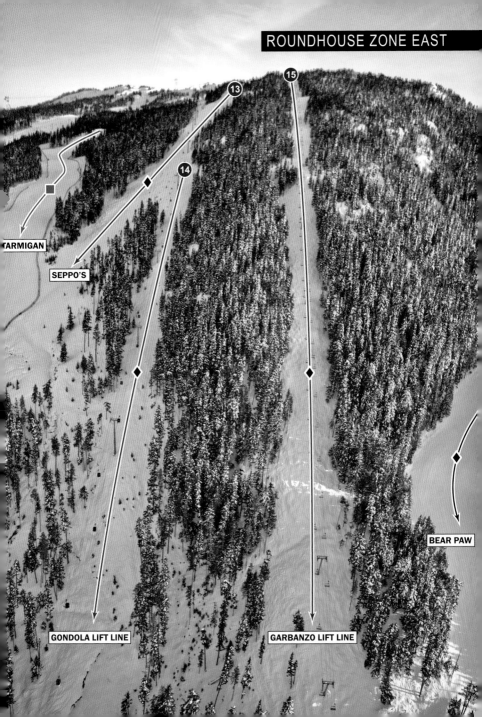

ROUNDHOUSE ZONE EAST

13

15

14

TARMIGAN

SEPPO'S

GONDOLA LIFT LINE

GARBANZO LIFT LINE

BEAR PAW

③ The Lower Glades

In the summer of 1999, Whistler Blackcomb thinned out some trees to create four new gladed runs on the lower mountain. Since these runs are at such low elevation, they rarely have good snow, but with the exception of Unsanctioned, they can be worth checking out if the snow gods provide.

⑯ Club 21 ♦ ★

Access via Raven. Look for the "Club 21" sign on the left and ride through the glades to Ptarmigan. If you want more of the same, take the skier's right variation, cross Ptarmigan and ride Side Order.

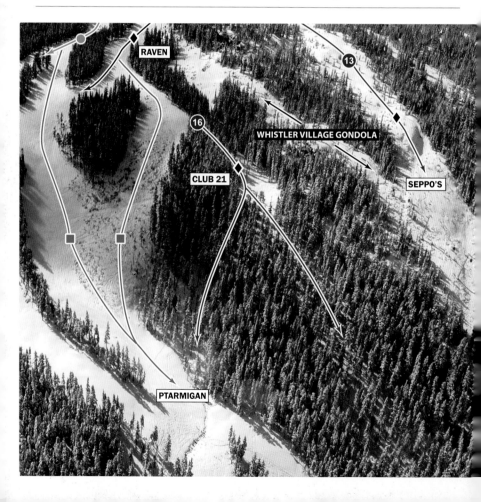

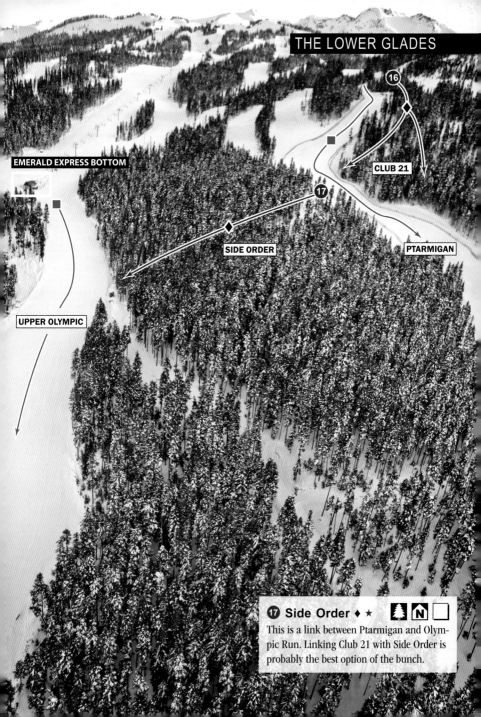

THE LOWER GLADES

16

CLUB 21

EMERALD EXPRESS BOTTOM

17

SIDE ORDER

PTARMIGAN

UPPER OLYMPIC

17 Side Order ♦ ★
This is a link between Ptarmigan and Olympic Run. Linking Club 21 with Side Order is probably the best option of the bunch.

18 Unsanctioned ♦

Quite possibly the worst run on Whistler. It's horribly off fall line and littered with exposed creek holes and fallen logs! Now you've gotta check it out, right? Access via Bear Paw.

19 In Deep ♦ ★

Access via Tokum.

Local's Tip

You've got to get pretty lucky to hit the Lower Glades in good conditions. They might be worth checking out if the following exist:

☐ There was more than 15 cm of new snow overnight.

☐ The valley air temperature is below 0° C.

☐ The mid-mountain base is over 200 cm.

☐ You've got an adventurous attitude.

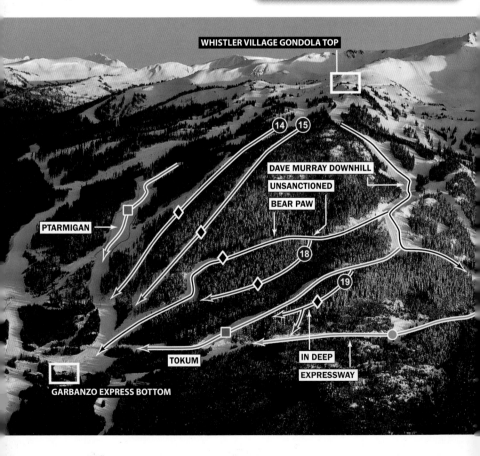

WHISTLER VILLAGE GONDOLA TOP

14 15

DAVE MURRAY DOWNHILL

UNSANCTIONED

BEAR PAW

PTARMIGAN

18

19

TOKUM

IN DEEP

EXPRESSWAY

GARBANZO EXPRESS BOTTOM

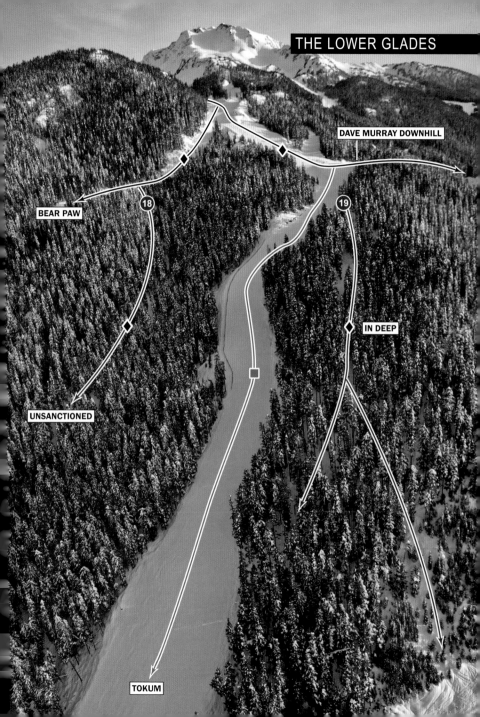

THE LOWER GLADES

DAVE MURRAY DOWNHILL

BEAR PAW

18

19

IN DEEP

UNSANCTIONED

TOKUM

④ T-Bar Zone

The two T-Bars on Whistler Mountain run parallel to one another and can be easily accessed from the Roundhouse Lodge via a well-marked cat track. All runs listed in the T-Bar section can be accessed by either the Harmony Express or the Peak Chair; however, they are listed here because the T-Bars are the lowest lifts allowing access.

⑳ T-Bar Bowl ♦ ★

This gentle slope makes for a nice warm-up.

㉑ Headwall ♦ ★★

Great terrain beside the T-bar. This is a good run to do a couple of times while awaiting an imminent Peak Chair opening. Access by a short hike from the start of the traverse to Ridge Run.

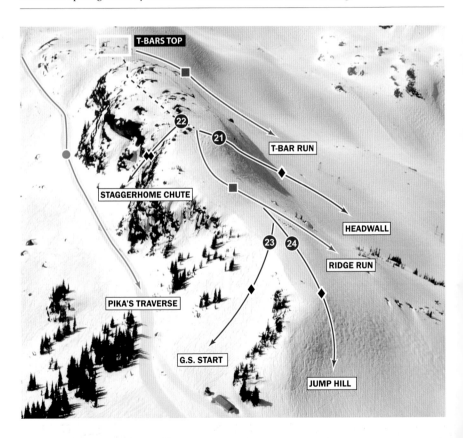

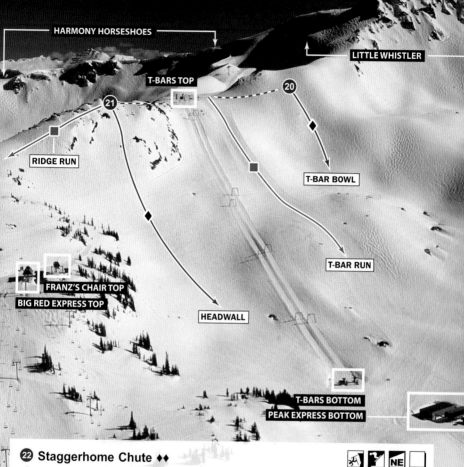

HARMONY HORSESHOES

LITTLE WHISTLER

T-BARS TOP

21

20

RIDGE RUN

T-BAR BOWL

T-BAR RUN

FRANZ'S CHAIR TOP

BIG RED EXPRESS TOP

HEADWALL

T-BARS BOTTOM

PEAK EXPRESS BOTTOM

22 Staggerhome Chute ♦♦

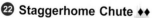

A very narrow chute accessed via Ridge Run.

23 G.S. Start ♦ ★

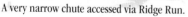

A short slope above Pika's Traverse, which is a nice approach to the Harmony Express. If you're headed to the lift, ride the gladed slope below the traverse and link up with G.S.

24 Jump Hill ♦ ★

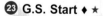

This steep little slope also makes for a good approach to Harmony. In the early '70s, this hill was the site of an annual Gelandesprung (ski jumping using alpine gear) competition, which earned the run its current moniker.

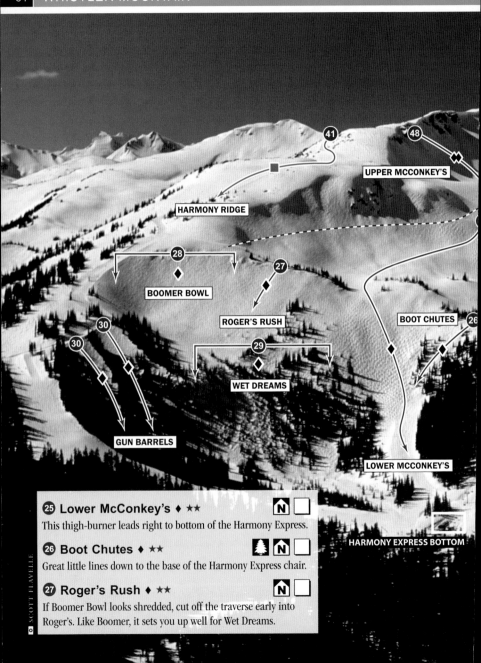

UPPER MCCONKEY'S

HARMONY RIDGE

BOOMER BOWL

ROGER'S RUSH

BOOT CHUTES

WET DREAMS

GUN BARRELS

LOWER MCCONKEY'S

HARMONY EXPRESS BOTTOM

25 Lower McConkey's ♦ ★★
This thigh-burner leads right to bottom of the Harmony Express.

26 Boot Chutes ♦ ★★
Great little lines down to the base of the Harmony Express chair.

27 Roger's Rush ♦ ★★
If Boomer Bowl looks shredded, cut off the traverse early into Roger's. Like Boomer, it sets you up well for Wet Dreams.

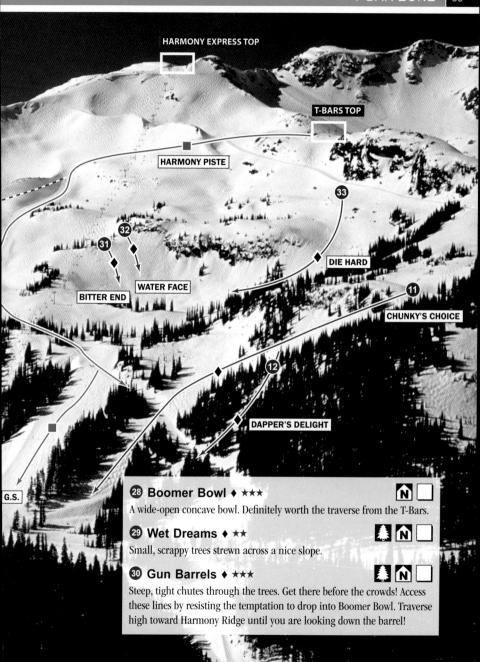

HARMONY EXPRESS TOP

T-BARS TOP

HARMONY PISTE

33

32

31

WATER FACE

DIE HARD

BITTER END

11

CHUNKY'S CHOICE

12

DAPPER'S DELIGHT

G.S.

28 Boomer Bowl ♦ ★★★

A wide-open concave bowl. Definitely worth the traverse from the T-Bars.

29 Wet Dreams ♦ ★★

Small, scrappy trees strewn across a nice slope.

30 Gun Barrels ♦ ★★★

Steep, tight chutes through the trees. Get there before the crowds! Access these lines by resisting the temptation to drop into Boomer Bowl. Traverse high toward Harmony Ridge until you are looking down the barrel!

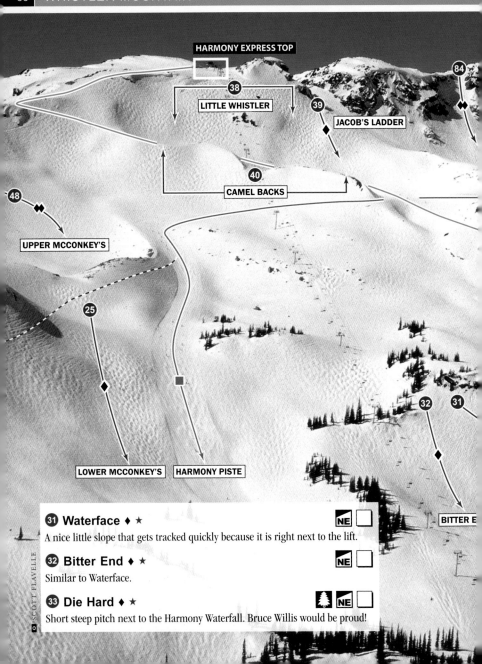

HARMONY EXPRESS TOP

84

38

LITTLE WHISTLER

39

JACOB'S LADDER

40

CAMEL BACKS

48

UPPER MCCONKEY'S

25

LOWER MCCONKEY'S   HARMONY PISTE

32   31

BITTER E

31 Waterface ♦ ★   **NE** ☐

A nice little slope that gets tracked quickly because it is right next to the lift.

32 Bitter End ♦ ★   **NE** ☐

Similar to Waterface.

33 Die Hard ♦ ★   🌲 **NE** ☐

Short steep pitch next to the Harmony Waterfall. Bruce Willis would be proud!

© SCOTT FLAVELLE

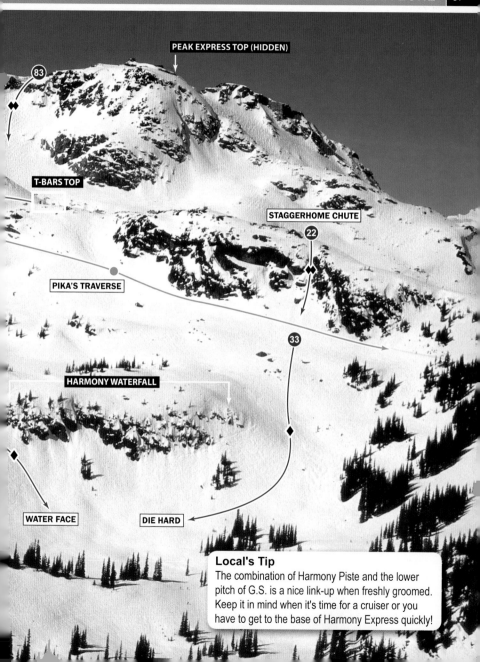

PEAK EXPRESS TOP (HIDDEN)

83

T-BARS TOP

STAGGERHOME CHUTE

22

PIKA'S TRAVERSE

33

HARMONY WATERFALL

WATER FACE

DIE HARD

Local's Tip
The combination of Harmony Piste and the lower pitch of G.S. is a nice link-up when freshly groomed. Keep it in mind when it's time for a cruiser or you have to get to the base of Harmony Express quickly!

⑤ Little Whistler

The installation of the Harmony Express chair in 1994 didn't open up any new terrain, but it changed the way everything got accessed. Prior to the lift, a trip out to Excitation or Little Whistler was a bit of a mission! Those days are over, and you now get whisked within steps of these great runs. Access Exhilaration, Excitation, Glacier Wall and Dilemma by hiking to the top of ridge, which is to your right as you get off the chair. There is often a well-worn bootpack to the ridge top.

㉞ Exhilaration ◆◆◆ ★★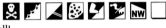
Very steep and narrow. Usually several humid storms must hit before it has adequate snow cover.

㉟ Excitation ◆◆ ★★★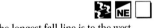
The best of the bunch. A steep, tight line designated by a rock pillar on the left. Mega!

㊱ Glacier Wall ◆◆◆ ★
Wait for adequate coverage before you put your balls to this wall!

㊲ Dilemma ◆◆◆ ★
A steep, interesting line.

㊳ Little Whistler ◆ ★★★
This classic lies directly underneath the upper section of the lift. The longest fall line is to the west.

㊴ Jacob's Ladder ◆ ★★
Sure, you loose a little vertical by traversing over to Jacob's, but it is often the last section that gets tracked out (and bumped up) by the masses.

㊵ Camel Backs ◆ ★
The large mounds split by the lift line. When linked with Little Whistler, they make a nice long run.

© SCOTT FLAVELLE (RIGHT)

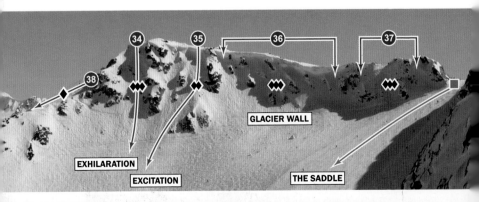

EXHILARATION
EXCITATION
GLACIER WALL
THE SADDLE

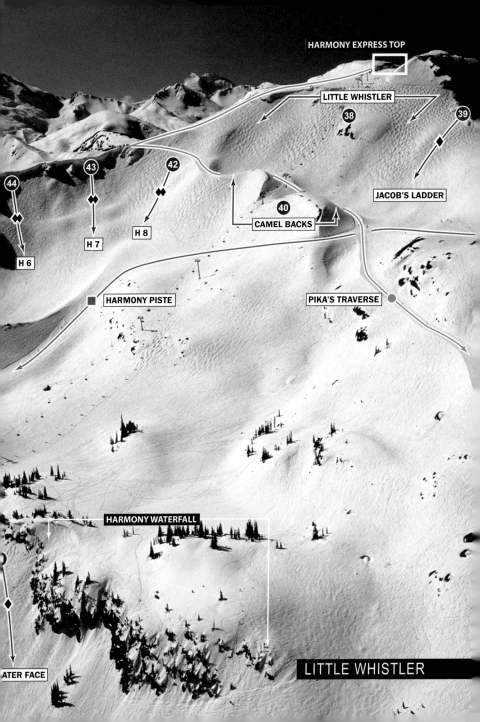

HARMONY EXPRESS TOP

LITTLE WHISTLER

38

39

JACOB'S LADDER

44

43

42

40

H 8

CAMEL BACKS

H 7

H 6

HARMONY PISTE

PIKA'S TRAVERSE

HARMONY WATERFALL

ATER FACE

LITTLE WHISTLER

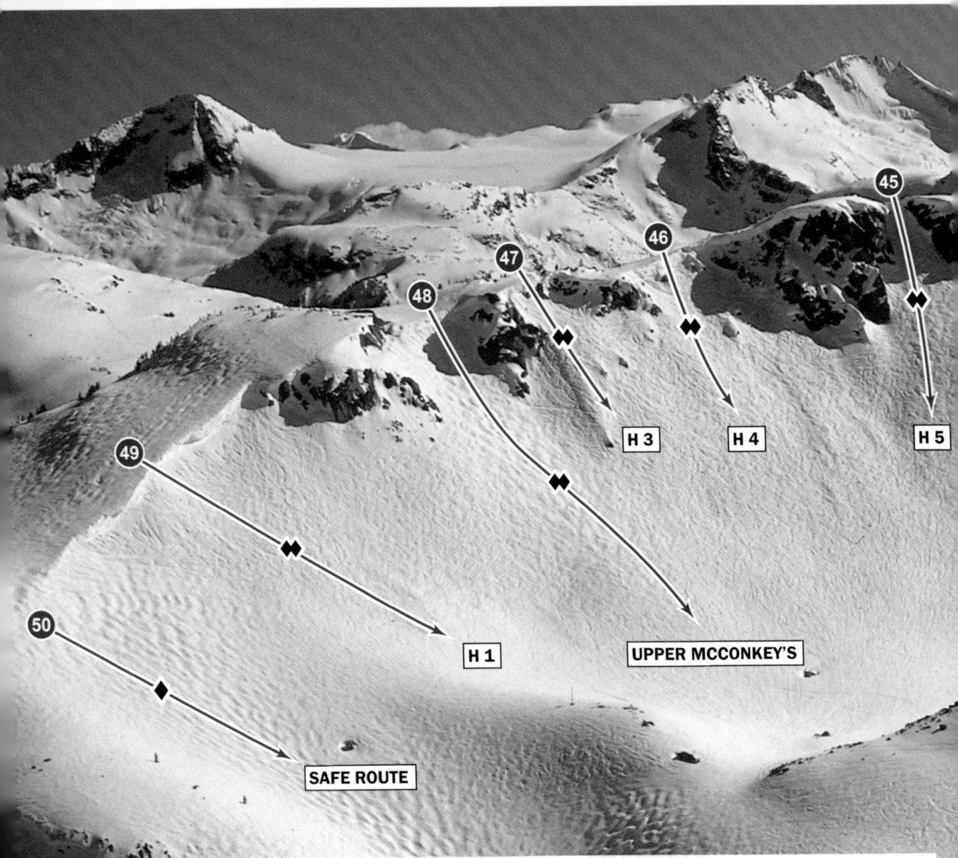
45
46
47
48
49
50
H 3
H 4
H 5
H 1
UPPER MCCONKEY'S
SAFE ROUTE

6 Harmony Ridge

This corniced ridge has several short chutes. All are accessed from the Harmony Ridge run.

---

41 Harmony Ridge ■

Consider this run your artery to some of the best terrain the Harmony Chair has to offer. Remember, you're sharing this run with skiers of all abilities.

42 Horseshoe 8 ♦♦ ★★

43 Horseshoe 7 ♦♦ ★★

44 Horseshoe 6 ♦♦ ★

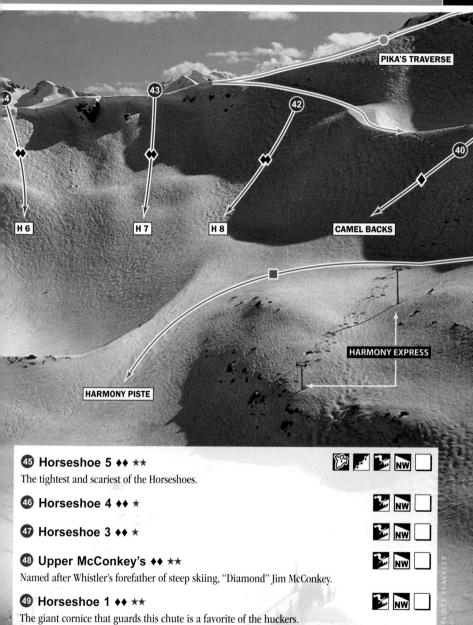

PIKA'S TRAVERSE

43

42

40

◆

◆ H 6

◆ H 7

◆ H 8

◆ CAMEL BACKS

HARMONY EXPRESS

HARMONY PISTE

45 **Horseshoe 5** ◆◆ ★★
The tightest and scariest of the Horseshoes.

46 **Horseshoe 4** ◆◆ ★

47 **Horseshoe 3** ◆◆ ★

48 **Upper McConkey's** ◆◆ ★★
Named after Whistler's forefather of steep skiing, "Diamond" Jim McConkey.

49 **Horseshoe 1** ◆◆ ★★
The giant cornice that guards this chute is a favorite of the huckers.

50 Safe Route ♦ ★

The first lower-angle slope leading off Harmony Ridge into Harmony Bowl. It connects nicely with a traverse over to Boomer Bowl or a descent of Lower McConkey's.

51 Low Roll ♦ ★

A good line that can be used to access Boomer Bowl and Wet Dreams.

52 KC Roll ♦♦ ★★

A very steep slope.

53 Kaleidoscope ♦ ★★

Similar to Low Roll, only better!

Local's Tip

As the moist, southwesterly storms rumble through the Whistler region throughout the winter, cornices slowly build on the north side of the ridges. The ski patrol wages a season-long war against these cornices as is evident by the bomb holes near the ridge tops. Savvy skiers learn to expect cornice chunks on the slopes below the ridges and are sure to remember them when the visibility is poor! Dive in with caution...

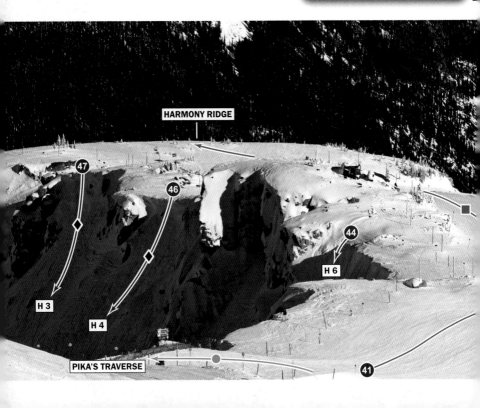

HARMONY RIDGE

47

46

44

H 6

H 3

H 4

PIKA'S TRAVERSE

41

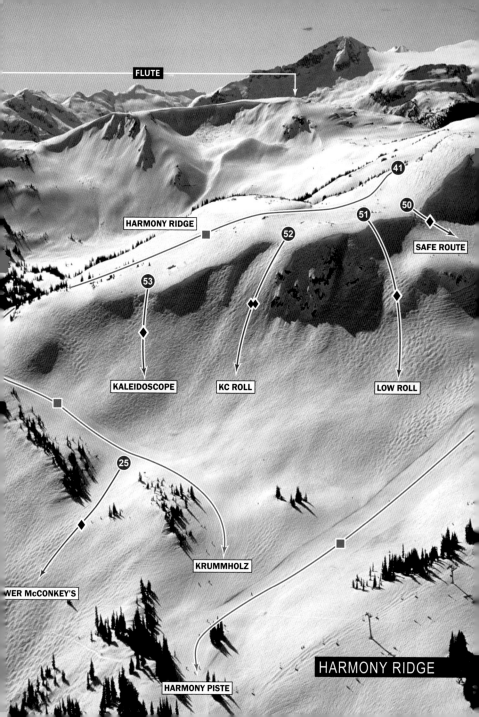

FLUTE

HARMONY RIDGE

41

51

50

SAFE ROUTE

52

53

KALEIDOSCOPE

KC ROLL

LOW ROLL

25

WER McCONKEY'S

KRUMMHOLZ

HARMONY PISTE

HARMONY RIDGE

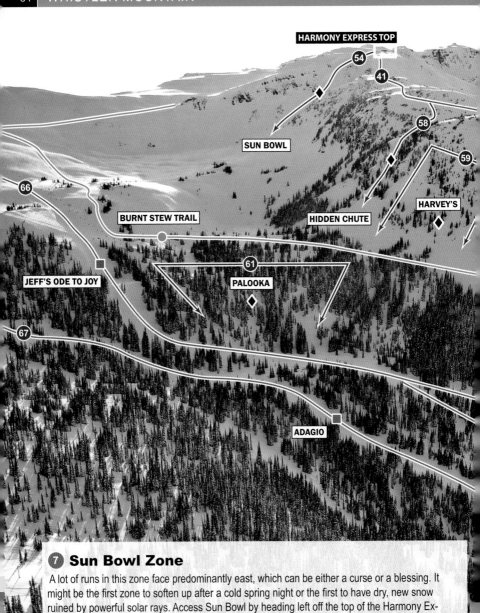

HARMONY EXPRESS TOP

54

41

58

SUN BOWL

59

66

BURNT STEW TRAIL

HARVEY'S

HIDDEN CHUTE

61

JEFF'S ODE TO JOY

PALOOKA

67

ADAGIO

⑦ Sun Bowl Zone

A lot of runs in this zone face predominantly east, which can be either a curse or a blessing. It might be the first zone to soften up after a cold spring night or the first to have dry, new snow ruined by powerful solar rays. Access Sun Bowl by heading left off the top of the Harmony Express chair. Almost immediately, you will see signs directing you (skier's right) to Sun Bowl.

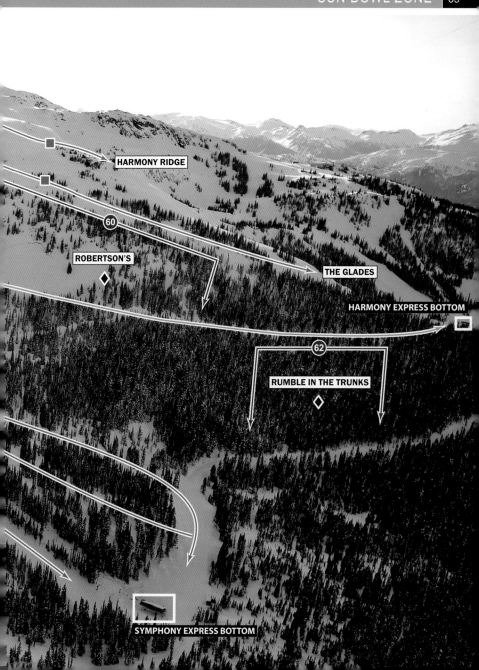

HARMONY RIDGE

60

ROBERTSON'S

THE GLADES

HARMONY EXPRESS BOTTOM

62

RUMBLE IN THE TRUNKS

SYMPHONY EXPRESS BOTTOM

54 Sun Bowl ♦ ★★

Great terrain and lots of it. Be sure to wear your shades!

55 Sun Bowl Chutes ♦♦ ★

Steep lines next to the main bowl.

56 Safe Route Chutes ♦ ★

These steep tree lines are accessed from Harmony Ridge (Blue), and skiers pursuing more visible runs often ignore them. Check 'em out if everything else is tracked.

57 Hourglass ♦ ★

Like snow through the hourglass, so are the days of our lives! This is a nice little powder stash that can be accessed from the Safe Route Chutes.

SUN BOWL

BURNT STEW TRAIL

HARMONY RIDGE

SUN BOWL CHUTES

SUN BOWL

58 Hidden Chute ♦ ★

A scrappy, off-fall-line diagonal run.

59 Harvey's Harrow ♦ ★★★

A classic, gladed slope with a consistent pitch. When the Symphony Express is open, you can ski Lower Harvey's below the Burnt Stew Trail to Jeff's Ode to Joy.

60 Robertson's Run ♦ ★★★

Great skiing through glades and well-spaced old-growth trees. Worth the traverse if Boomer Bowl is tracked! As with Harvey's, you can extend your run and ride down to the Symphony chair if it's open.

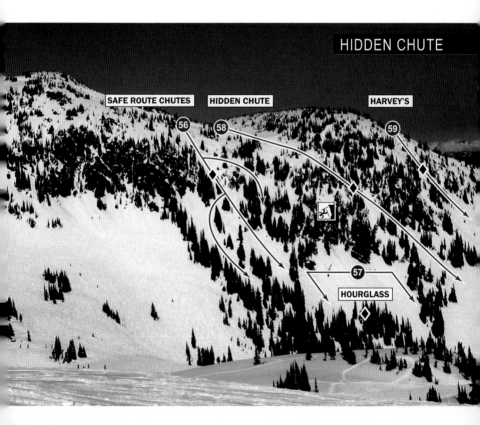

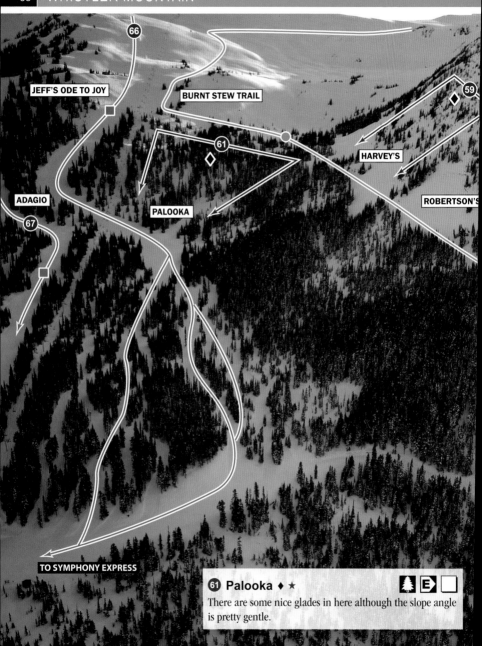

66

JEFF'S ODE TO JOY

BURNT STEW TRAIL

59

61

HARVEY'S

ADAGIO

67

PALOOKA

ROBERTSON'S

TO SYMPHONY EXPRESS

61 Palooka ♦ ★

There are some nice glades in here although the slope angle is pretty gentle.

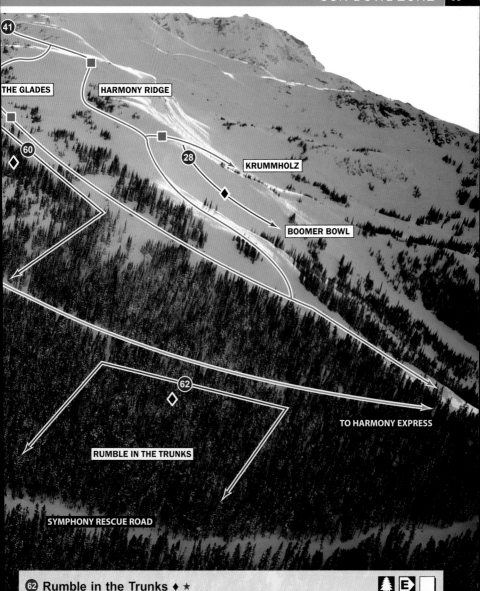

THE GLADES

HARMONY RIDGE

KRUMMHOLZ

BOOMER BOWL

TO HARMONY EXPRESS

RUMBLE IN THE TRUNKS

SYMPHONY RESCUE ROAD

62 Rumble in the Trunks ♦ ★

This short pitch with nicely spaced trees lies between Burnt Stew Road and the access road to Symphony. Make sure the lift is open before skiing it and don't ski below the road; it's out of bounds.

⑧ Symphony Zone

The Symphony Express chair opened in December 2006 and although it primarily services intermediate terrain, the chair provides quick circuits on Piccolo and Flute for the experts, all with incredible views! The Symphony Express unloads on the ridge below the summit of a minor peak called Piccolo. Although short, the north aspect of Piccolo offers up some exciting terrain.

Access: From the top of the Harmony Express, ride the Burnt Stew Trail into Symphony Bowl. Continue along this run until you see a junction, leading to the right near Tower 15 of the Symphony Express. From this point, ski Jeff's Ode to Joy to the base of the chair.

Egress: All runs lead back to the base of the Symphony Express. To exit from the Symphony Amphitheatre, ride the chair up and ski down Jeff's Ode to Joy to the point where it intersects with Burnt Stew Trail near Tower 13. From here, ride Burnt Stew back to the Harmony Express. It is important to realize that the elevation of the bottom of the Symphony Express is much lower than that of Harmony Express. Therefore, if you miss the last chair, it will cost you a half-hour hike up the Symphony Rescue Road to get to lower Harmony Ridge and descend to the bottom of the Harmony Express.

---

⑥③ Piccolo North Face ♦♦ ★★

Turn right after getting off the chair and sneak your way through the rocks to access this steep, varied slope.

⑥④ Summit Slope ♦♦ ★★

Access as for the North Face, then traverse under the summit of Piccolo.

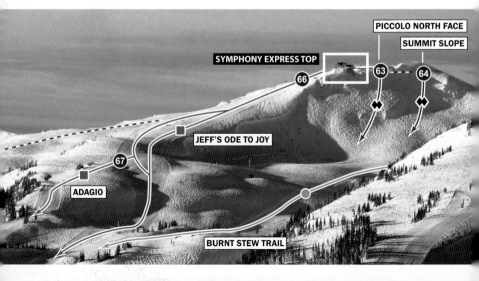

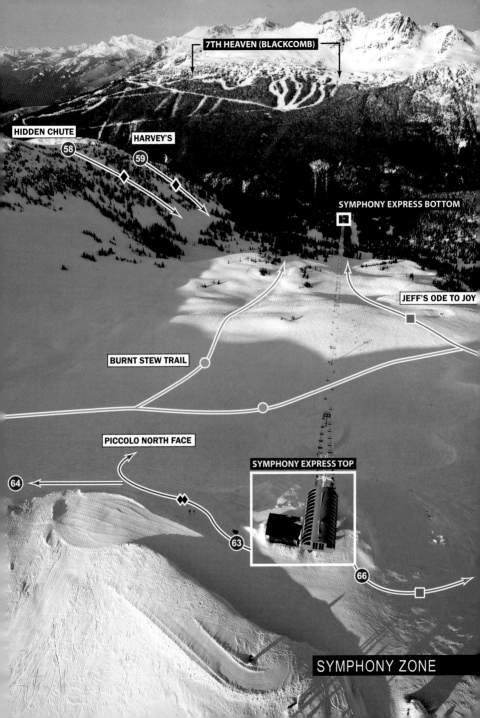

7TH HEAVEN (BLACKCOMB)

HIDDEN CHUTE
58

HARVEY'S
59

SYMPHONY EXPRESS BOTTOM

JEFF'S ODE TO JOY

BURNT STEW TRAIL

PICCOLO NORTH FACE

64

SYMPHONY EXPRESS TOP

63

66

SYMPHONY ZONE

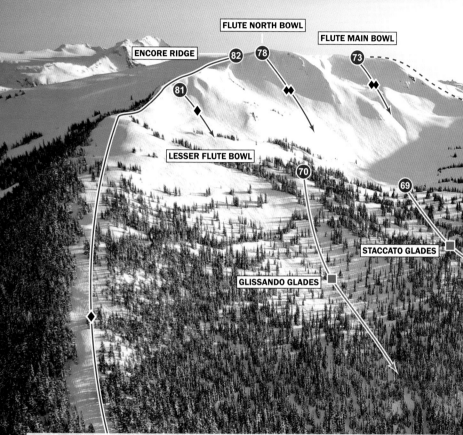

FLUTE NORTH BOWL

FLUTE MAIN BOWL

ENCORE RIDGE

82 **78** **73**

81

LESSER FLUTE BOWL

70

69

STACCATO GLADES

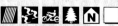
GLISSANDO GLADES

65 Piccolo Main ♦ ★★

Traverse across the top of Summit Slope to access. This line sets you up really well for continuing past the Burnt Stew Trail and onto a nice powder slope in Symphony Bowl.

66 Jeff's Ode to Joy ■ ★★

This low-angle cruiser is the main access route to the base of the lift. Islands of trees have been preserved to provide a more "gladed" feel on the final pitches. The patrol calls these glades the Founder's Fingers since Jeff's Ode to Joy is also known as Founder's Run.

67 Adagio ■ ★★

The word "adagio" is Italian for "at ease", and it's a fitting name for this serene groomer.

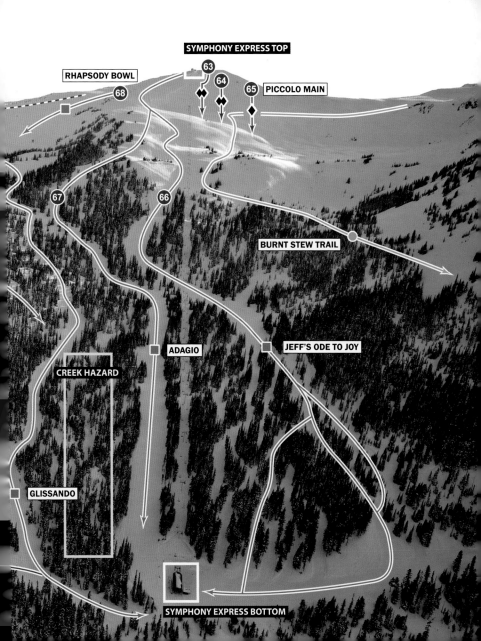

SYMPHONY EXPRESS TOP

63

RHAPSODY BOWL

68

64

65 PICCOLO MAIN

67

66

BURNT STEW TRAIL

ADAGIO

JEFF'S ODE TO JOY

CREEK HAZARD

GLISSANDO

SYMPHONY EXPRESS BOTTOM

68 Rhapsody Bowl (formerly Boundary Bowl) ■ ★★

When the visibility is poor in the high alpine, don't forget about Boundary Bowl. There are just enough trees flanking the bowl to provide reference in flat light.

69 Staccato Glades ■

If "staccato" were Italian for "flat," then this run would be appropriately named.

70 Glissando Glades ■

There are a few good turns to be had in here, but overall the terrain is pretty flat for powder skiing. Some of the better lines in Glissando descend from Encore ridge, but this is a long walk for a few turns. If you are a serious powderhound willing to work for those last bits of powder remaining on the hill, then this run is for you.

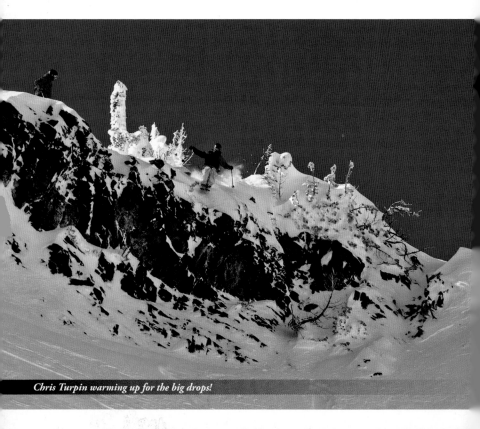

Chris Turpin warming up for the big drops!

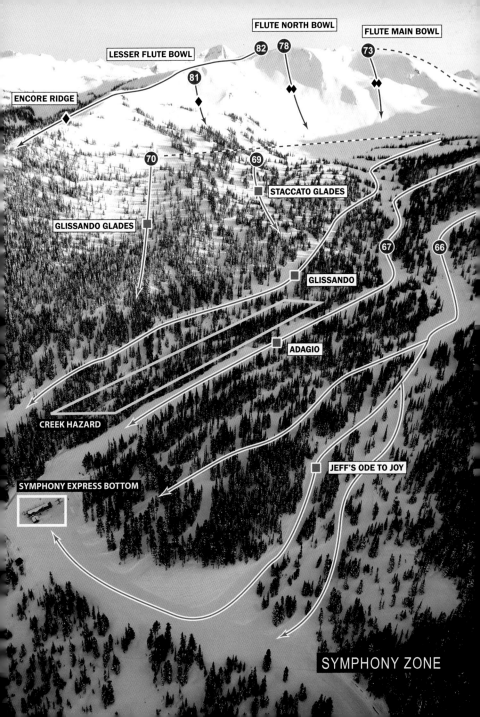

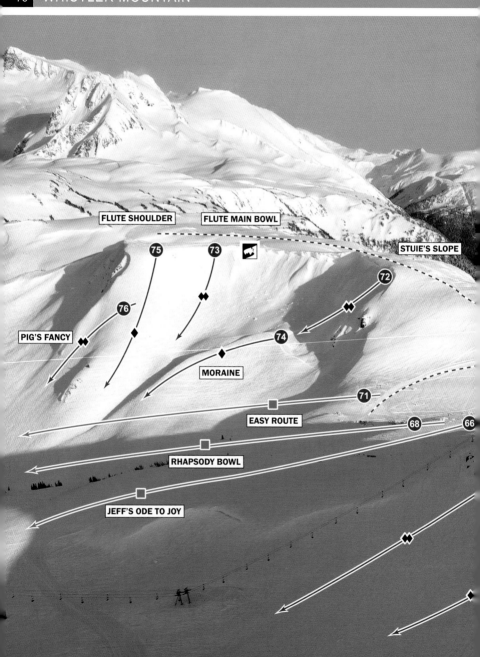

FLUTE SHOULDER

FLUTE MAIN BOWL

STUIE'S SLOPE

75

73

72

76

PIG'S FANCY

74

MORAINE

71

EASY ROUTE

68

66

RHAPSODY BOWL

JEFF'S ODE TO JOY

⑨ Flute

Flute sits on the border to Garibaldi Provincial Park, forming the highest point on the Musical Bumps ridge. All but the Easy Route require hiking up a thigh-burning groomed track, but gaining access to steep, north-facing terrain like this makes it well worth the effort. The area receives avalanche control and ski patrol attention but maintains its remote feel because grooming is limited to the ascent route and the track out from the base of the peak.

Access: Flute is best accessed from the top of the Symphony Express. From here, ski into the saddle between Piccolo and Flute and locate the groomed up-track leading to the summit. You have to earn it from here!

Egress: Locate the groomed track (marked with fluorescent discs mounted on bamboo poles) at the base of Flute. This track will lead you back to the bottom of the Symphony Express. Remember, if you don't get back to the base of Symphony before it closes, you have to walk up the rescue road to get to Harmony Ridge and descend to the bottom of the Harmony Express. This will take you about 30 minutes from the base of Symphony.

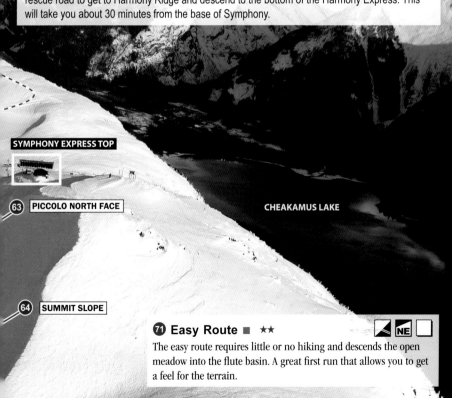

SYMPHONY EXPRESS TOP

㊿ PICCOLO NORTH FACE

CHEAKAMUS LAKE

㉔ SUMMIT SLOPE

㉛ Easy Route ■ ★★

The easy route requires little or no hiking and descends the open meadow into the flute basin. A great first run that allows you to get a feel for the terrain.

72 Stuie's Slope ♦♦ ★★

A steep face leading into the main bowl. Stuie's is named for a Whistler local who was killed in an avalanche on this slope. Sadly, this is one of the few ways to have a run named after you.

73 Flute Main Bowl ♦♦ ★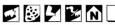

The main bowl, although good, is often littered with avalanche debris and requires you to navigate (or ski under) a burly cornice to access. Watch out!

74 Moraine ♦ ★

Access from Stuie's, or if you're a slacker, save yourself the hike to the top and traverse in from the west ridge.

75 Flute Shoulder ♦ ★★★

The shoulder is probably the best bang for your buck; it is the longest ski run at a consistent grade in the Flute Area. Don't miss it!

76 Pig's Fancy ♦♦ ★★★

Although not the steepest line in the area, this gem catches the best powder of any line in the Flute area. Find your way onto the shoulder and break off skiers right onto the steeper slope. If you get there first, don't stop until you get to the bottom; it could be the run of your life!

77 Flute Chutes ♦♦♦ ★★

A steep and intimidating start leads to stellar, open bowl riding!

78 Flute North Bowl ♦♦ ★★★

The entire North Bowl offers great powder skiing and is usually last to get shredded because of the long hike up.

Local's Tip

A great way to ski Flute is to descend Flute Shoulder directly to the little patch of trees that is visible in the photo. At the trees, stop and give your legs a rest before skiing the nice, planar slope below to the cat track leading back to the Symphony Express. This makes for an exhilarating, fall line run!

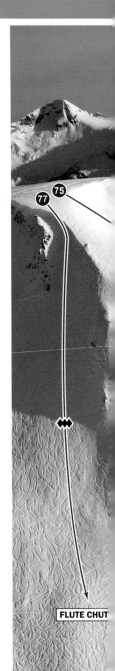

FLUTE CHUT

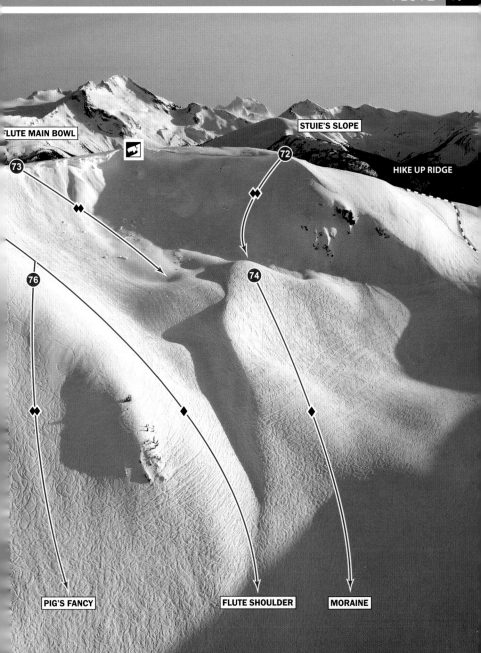

FLUTE MAIN BOWL

STUIE'S SLOPE

HIKE UP RIDGE

73

72

76

74

PIG'S FANCY

FLUTE SHOULDER

MORAINE

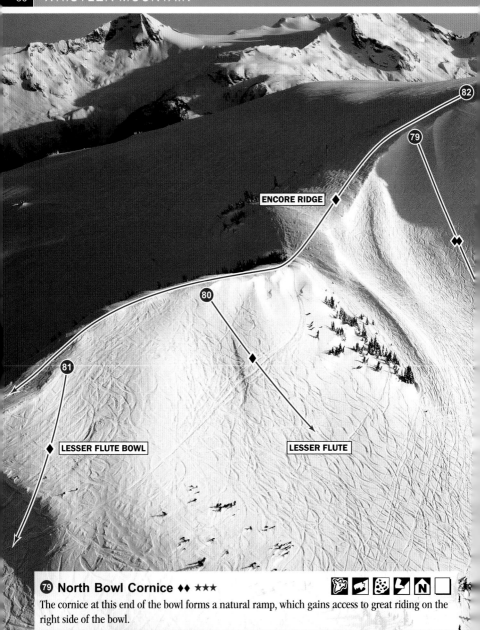

82

79

ENCORE RIDGE

80

81

LESSER FLUTE BOWL

LESSER FLUTE

79 North Bowl Cornice ♦♦ ★★★

The cornice at this end of the bowl forms a natural ramp, which gains access to great riding on the right side of the bowl.

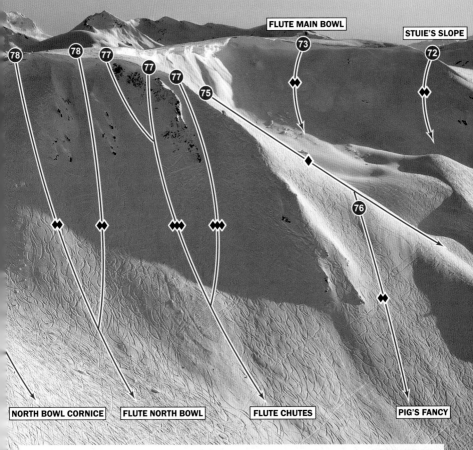

FLUTE MAIN BOWL

STUIE'S SLOPE

NORTH BOWL CORNICE   FLUTE NORTH BOWL   FLUTE CHUTES   PIG'S FANCY

80 Lesser Flute ♦ ★

Lower-angled skiing through a series of tree islands, reminiscent of a classic heli-ski run.

81 Lesser Flute Bowl ♦ ★

This is a smaller bowl on the east end of the series of bowls that offers great lines. The walk is a little longer, but those seeking to get away from the crowds won't be disappointed.

82 Encore Ridge ♦

This is really just a run to define the ski-area boundary. To access Encore, you have to hike up and over Flute and Lesser Flute to reach this flat, wind-hammered ridge. It takes about 40 minutes to earn the 23 turns that Encore Ridge provides! Trust us, no one will be asking for an encore!

⑩ Glacier Bowl

The Peak Chair is arguably the best lift on the continent for spinning laps on steep alpine terrain. It is the principal lift for accessing Whistler Bowl, West Bowl, Bagel Bowl and Glacier Bowl, the latter of which is an awesome wind-protected bowl with several entry options. To access Glacier Bowl, head left off the top of the chair and glide along Matthew's Traverse until you see a sign directing you (skier's left) to the run of your choice. All lines can be ridden back to the bottom of the Peak Chair!

㉜ The Cirque ♦♦ ★★★

Negotiate your way down an ugly, rocky ramp to what is often the most wind-protected section of Glacier Bowl.

㉝ The Couloir ♦♦ ★★★

Steep skiing into the heart of the bowl. A local's favorite.

㉞ The Saddle ■ ★★

The ski area has gone to great lengths to open the Saddle up to the intermediate rider. Blasting at the ridge-top has created a more open entrance and allowed for regular grooming.

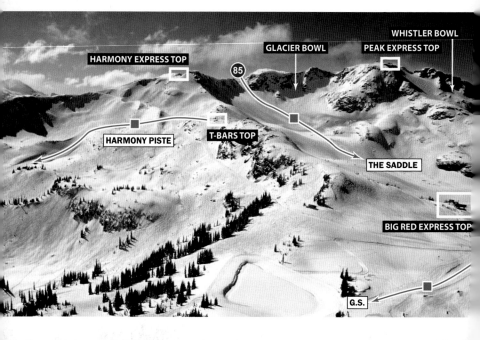

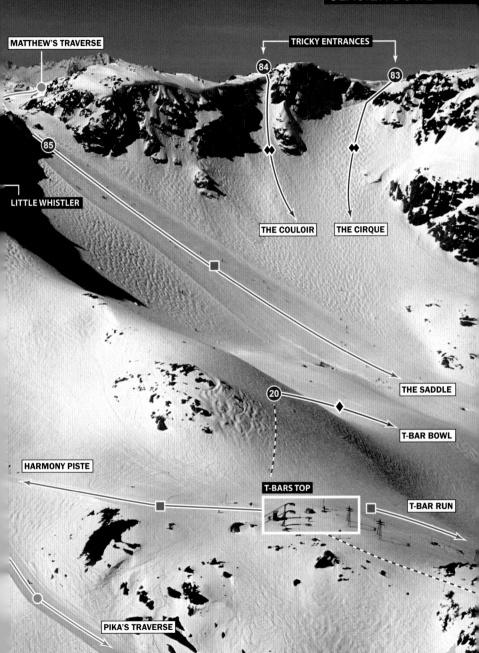

GLACIER BOWL

MATTHEW'S TRAVERSE

TRICKY ENTRANCES

84

83

85

LITTLE WHISTLER

THE COULOIR

THE CIRQUE

THE SADDLE

20

T-BAR BOWL

HARMONY PISTE

T-BARS TOP

T-BAR RUN

PIKA'S TRAVERSE

⑪ Whistler Bowl

Classic, wide-open alpine terrain.

㊏ Whistler Cornice ♦♦ ★★

As you approach the top of the chair, look to your left. You will see a cellular tower on top of the mound. On the other side of the mound from the chair is the entrance to Whistler Cornice. The east side of the bowl, which this run will set you up for, has a beautiful fall line and often fewer moguls.

㊐ Liftie's Leap ♦♦ ★★

A steep little roll behind the top lift shack. This run is named after Len Letain, a former lift operator from Winnipeg (of all places).

㊑ Whistler Bowl Main Entrance ♦ ★★★

The widest-open access to the bowl. This entrance will set you up best for a descent down the heart of the bowl.

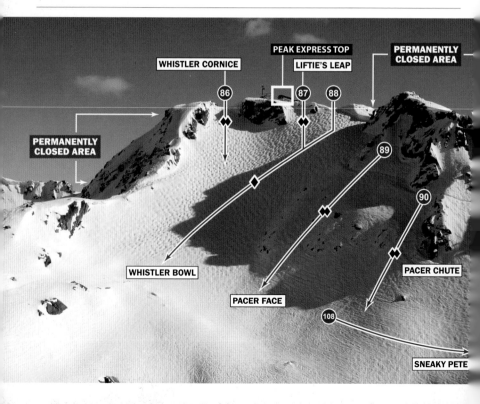

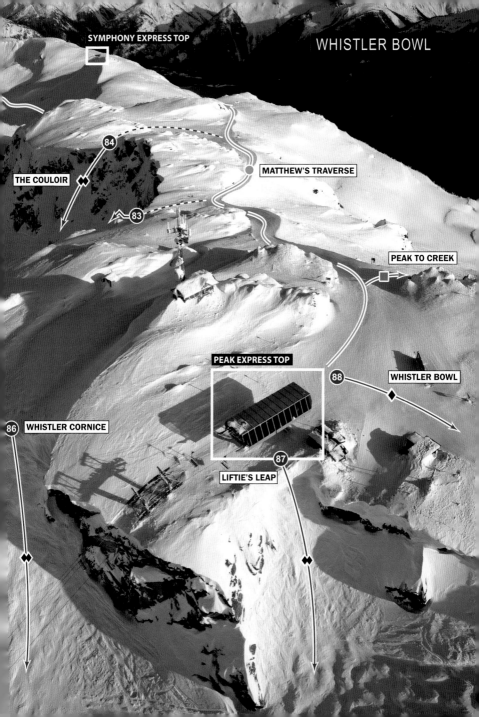

SYMPHONY EXPRESS TOP

WHISTLER BOWL

84

THE COULOIR

83

MATTHEW'S TRAVERSE

PEAK TO CREEK

PEAK EXPRESS TOP

88

WHISTLER BOWL

86

WHISTLER CORNICE

87

LIFTIE'S LEAP

89 Pacer Face ♦♦ ★★

A steep, convex face. Traverse in from Whistler Bowl Main Entrance.

90 Pacer Chute ♦♦ ★★

A steep, fall-line shot.

91 West Cirque ♦♦ ★★★

Mega-classic steep face. Access the line by following Upper Peak to Creek to a junction with a cat track known as John Glenn Road (on your right). Follow John Glenn Road to the Permanent Closure fence above West Bowl. Hike up along the fence line, back toward Whistler Bowl. Trust us—it's worth it! See photo on page 100 for access.

92 Doom and Gloom ♦ ★★★

This ironically named run is so good it could put Prozac out of business! Great terrain that is often neglected for more prominent lines.

93 Grande Finale ♦ ★★

The name says it all. A classy finish to Whistler Bowl.

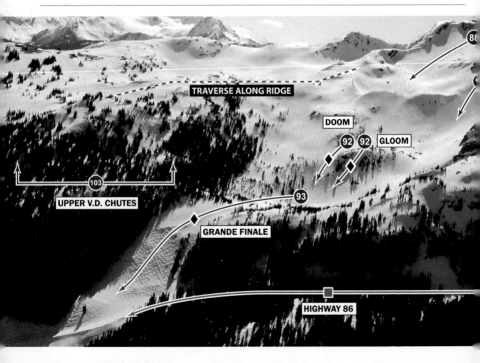

TRAVERSE ALONG RIDGE

DOOM

92 92 GLOOM

103

UPPER V.D. CHUTES

93

GRANDE FINALE

HIGHWAY 86

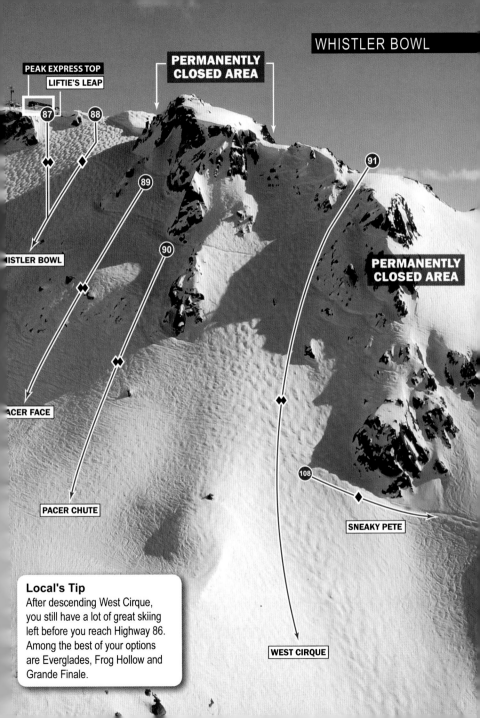

WHISTLER BOWL

PERMANENTLY CLOSED AREA

PEAK EXPRESS TOP

LIFTIE'S LEAP

87

88

91

89

90

PERMANENTLY CLOSED AREA

ISTLER BOWL

ACER FACE

PACER CHUTE

108

SNEAKY PETE

WEST CIRQUE

Local's Tip
After descending West Cirque, you still have a lot of great skiing left before you reach Highway 86. Among the best of your options are Everglades, Frog Hollow and Grande Finale.

⑫ Lower Peak Chair Zone

The beauty of this zone is that all of the runs except Tigers Terrace and Upper VD Chutes will deposit you back at the base of the Peak Chair. Access to this zone is via Whistler Bowl.

㉔ Surprise ♦ ★★★

Awesome varied terrain. Bet you can't ride it the same way twice! To get to this run, stay skier's right in upper Whistler Bowl and look for the "Surprise" signs directing you to pass under the Peak Chair lift line.

㉕ North Face Low ♦ ★★

A cool little drop under the Peak Chair lift line.

㉖ Chris's Drop ♦ ★★

A great pitch that is often left untracked in favor of the more open Shale Slope. There are some fun little cliffs and rocks to jump off here too.

㉗ Shale Slope ♦ ★★★

A true Whistler icon. After skiing the main slope of Whistler Bowl, head to the skier's right and look for the signs directing you to Shale Slope. Use the Whistler Bowl overview photo as your guide.

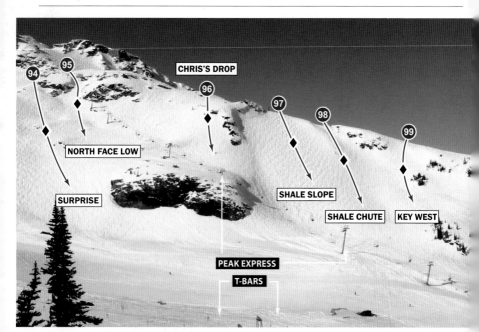

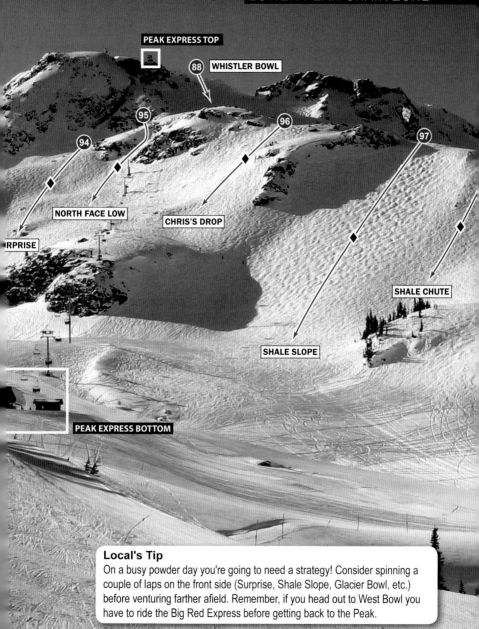

PEAK EXPRESS TOP

88 WHISTLER BOWL

95

94

NORTH FACE LOW

CHRIS'S DROP

96

97

SHALE CHUTE

RPRISE

SHALE SLOPE

PEAK EXPRESS BOTTOM

Local's Tip
On a busy powder day you're going to need a strategy! Consider spinning a couple of laps on the front side (Surprise, Shale Slope, Glacier Bowl, etc.) before venturing farther afield. Remember, if you head out to West Bowl you have to ride the Big Red Express before getting back to the Peak.

98 Shale Chute ♦ ★★

Sometimes, due to the convexity of the terrain, the snow is a little more wind protected than it is on Shale Slope.

99 Key West ♦ ★★

This line receives much less traffic than Shale Slope and, therefore, develops fewer moguls.

100 Left Hook ♦ ★★

Gladed run beside Shale Slope. If you don't hook left, you'll be set up for a launch off the Waterfall!

101 Tiger's Terrace ♦ ★★

Short but sweet tree lines. Often left alone by the hordes. After all, this is tiger country! Access this area by continuing along the ridge from the top of Shale Slope.

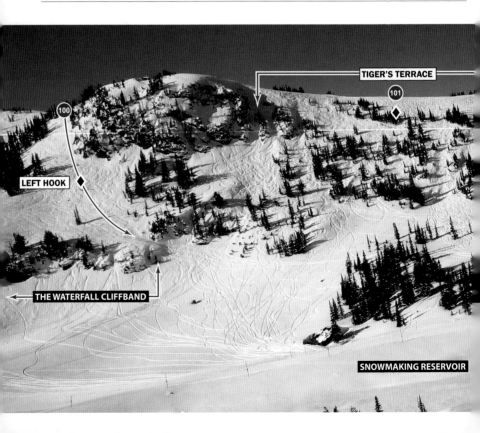

Interesting Fact
There is a bronze plaque affixed to one of the boulders on the ridge in the photo below. The plaque was placed as a memorial to Sean Walsh, a longtime Whistler ski patroller who was tragically killed while performing avalanche control.

102 Come Chute ♦♦

A steep chute above Franz's Meadow.

103 Upper V.D. Chutes ♦♦ ★

Good glade skiing. Continue down the ridge above Tiger's Terrace and choose a line heading either down to Grand Finale or fall line to Highway 86.

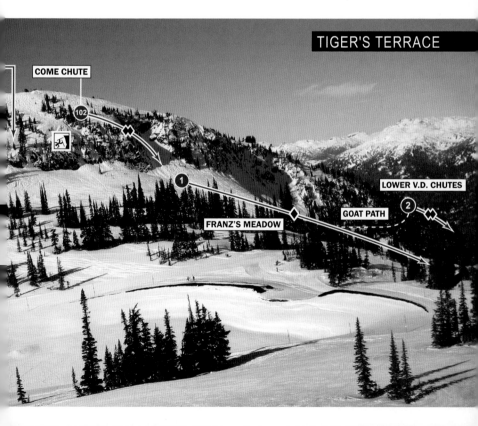

TIGER'S TERRACE

COME CHUTE

102

LOWER V.D. CHUTES

2

GOAT PATH

FRANZ'S MEADOW

1

⑬ West Ridge Zone

West Ridge is the ridge that divides Whistler Bowl and West Bowl. Access the ridge by taking Sneaky Pete's traverse from Whistler Bowl. The traverse will take you under Pacer Face and West Cirque to the top of West Ridge. Being cautious of cliffs on either side of the ridge, slide along the crest of West Ridge from the top of Sneaky Pete to access the runs below.

⑩④ Sunrise ◆◆ ★★

A steep little chute that gets the morning sun.

⑩⑤ Elevator ◆◆ ★

A very rocky line. It takes a lot of coverage before you can get any love in this elevator!

⑩⑥ Escalator ◆ ★★

Going down!

⑩⑦ Frog Hollow ◆ ★★

Good tree skiing to Highway 86. Access by riding to the end of West Ridge from the top of Sneaky Pete.

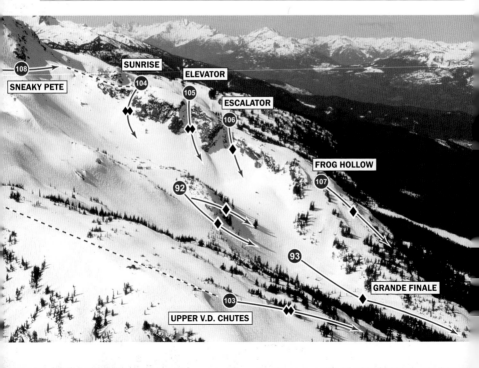

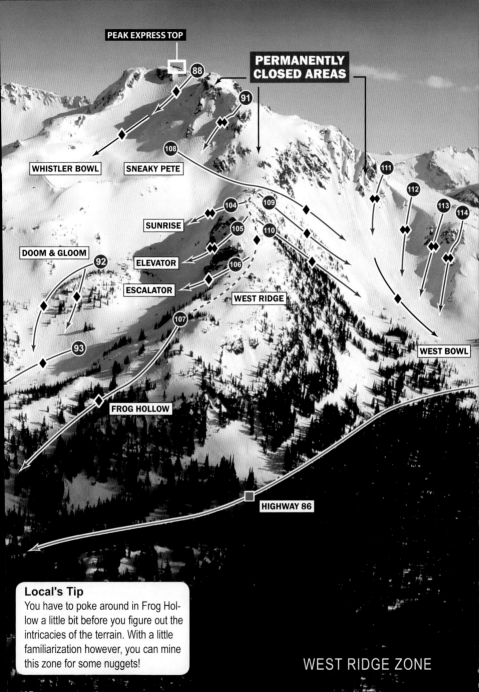

PEAK EXPRESS TOP

88

PERMANENTLY CLOSED AREAS

91

108

WHISTLER BOWL   SNEAKY PETE

111

112

113   114

104   109

SUNRISE

105   110

DOOM & GLOOM

92

ELEVATOR   106

ESCALATOR   WEST RIDGE

107

93

WEST BOWL

FROG HOLLOW

HIGHWAY 86

Local's Tip
You have to poke around in Frog Hollow a little bit before you figure out the intricacies of the terrain. With a little familiarization however, you can mine this zone for some nuggets!

WEST RIDGE ZONE

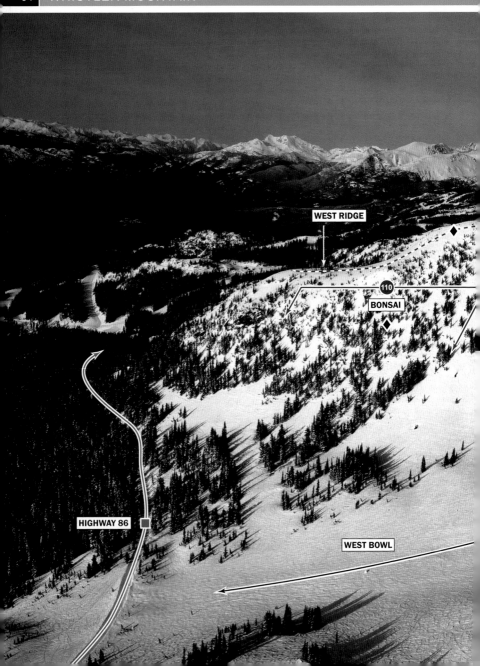

WEST RIDGE

110

BONSAI

HIGHWAY 86

WEST BOWL

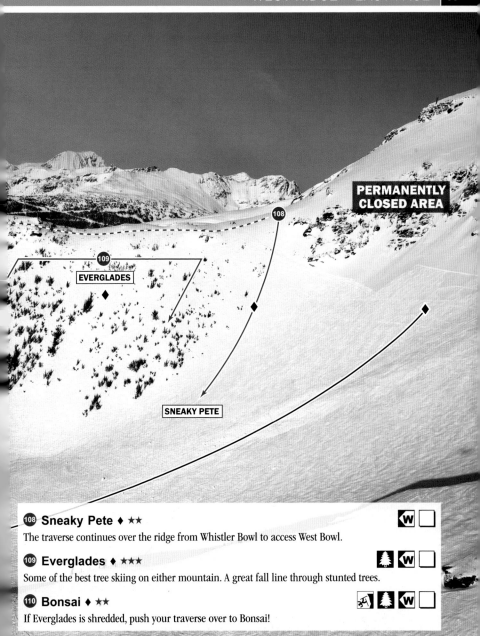

PERMANENTLY CLOSED AREA

108

109

EVERGLADES

SNEAKY PETE

108 Sneaky Pete ♦ ★★   W ☐

The traverse continues over the ridge from Whistler Bowl to access West Bowl.

109 Everglades ♦ ★★★   🌲 W ☐

Some of the best tree skiing on either mountain. A great fall line through stunted trees.

110 Bonsai ♦ ★★   🎿 🌲 W ☐

If Everglades is shredded, push your traverse over to Bonsai!

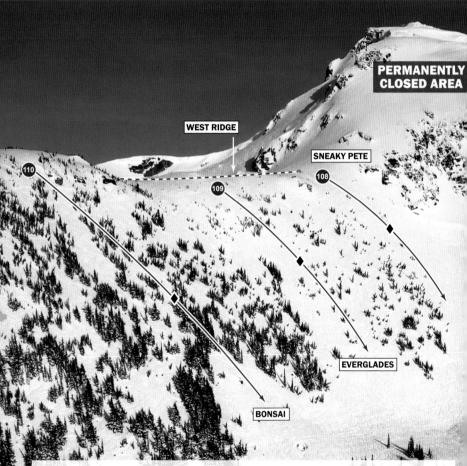

PERMANENTLY
CLOSED AREA

WEST RIDGE

SNEAKY PETE

110

109

108

EVERGLADES

BONSAI

14 West Bowl

An amazing expanse of alpine terrain. Access the bowl by taking Upper Peak to Creek past its junction with John Glenn Road (photo on page 100). After this point, on your right, will be a wind-scoured mass of crumbly rock. Slide over toward West Bowl around the downhill side of this rock.

111 Monday's ♦♦ ★★★

The highest legal entrance into West Bowl. This is one manic Monday!

112 Cockalorum ♦♦ ★★

This line often requires launching off a burly cornice.

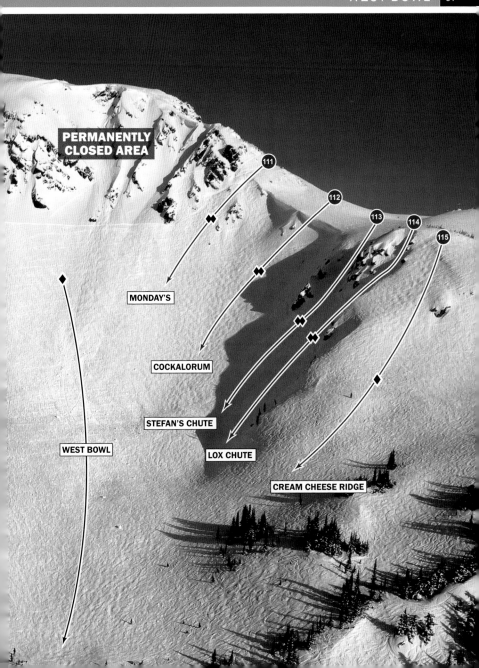

PERMANENTLY CLOSED AREA

111

112

113

114

115

MONDAY'S

COCKALORUM

STEFAN'S CHUTE

WEST BOWL

LOX CHUTE

CREAM CHEESE RIDGE

⑬ Stefan's Chute ♦♦ ★★★
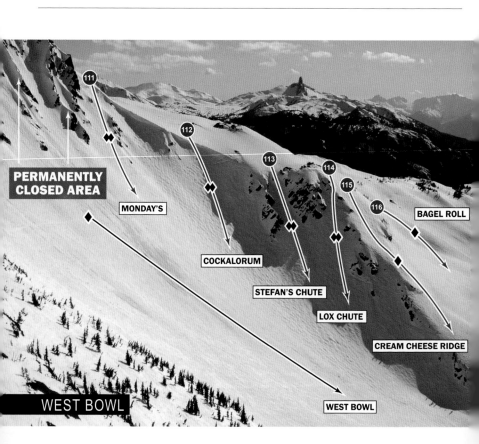
A classic, steep line that drops into the bowl.

⑭ Lox Chute ♦♦ ★★★
Very similar to Stefan's.

⑮ Cream Cheese Ridge ♦ ★★
Great varied terrain. Easier access to West Bowl than the chutes above.

⑯ Bagel Roll ♦ ★★★
This steep, convex roll between West Bowl and Bagel Bowl sets you up nicely to enter the glades above Highway 86. A great run.

Local's Tip
The steepness and due north exposure of Stefan's and Lox Chute allow for the preservation of cold, dry snow even after intense spring rays have had their way with neighboring slopes.

117 Bagel Bowl ♦ ★★   NW ☐
Good terrain, although it offers significantly less vertical for your effort.

118 Bernie's Bumps ♦ ★ NW ☐
A few interesting rolls, but pretty lame terrain overall. Sorry, Bernie!

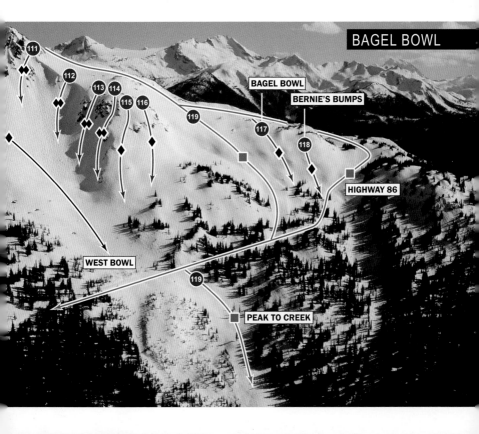

BAGEL BOWL

⑮ Peak to Creek

An expansion in 2004 opened up 1,100 acres of west-facing terrain on Whistler Mountain. All runs in the Peak to Creek zone are accessed via the Peak Express chair. You can ski any of the West Bowl runs into this area or you can follow Upper Peak to Creek from the top of the chair. All of the runs in the zone funnel into the bottom of the Creekside Gondola.

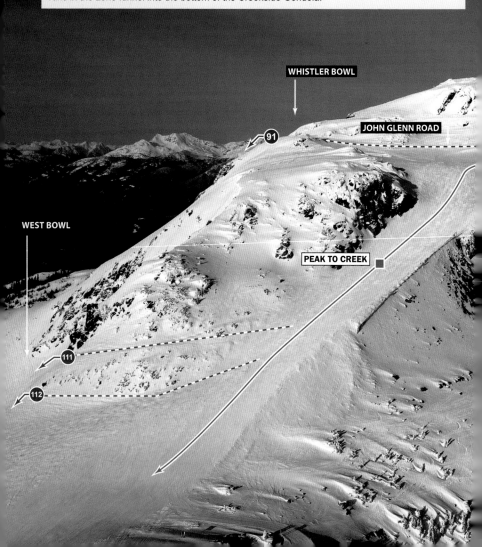

WHISTLER BOWL

JOHN GLENN ROAD

91

WEST BOWL

PEAK TO CREEK

111

112

119 **Peak to Creek** ■ ★★★

This is the jewel of the multimillion-dollar expansion. When freshly groomed, Peak to Creek is an amazing 1,530-metre (5,020-foot) descent from the alpine into the valley. I hope you've been following your Legs of Steel program!

PEAK EXPRESS TOP

119

MATTHEW'S TRAVERSE

OUT OF BOUNDS

OUT OF BOUNDS

Important Note
Peak to Creek is usually only groomed about twice a week below Highway 86! Make sure you are aware of the grooming status before committing to the full length of the run. When ungroomed, it can be an endless matrix of moguls and is certainly a black-diamond run in these conditions.

120 Big Timber ♦ ★

Unlike Peak to Creek, all of the natural rolls, drops and bushes have been left on this rugged descent. Consider it an adventure.

121 Dusty's Descent ♦ ★

Shorter than Big Timber, Dusty's allows you to get onto some rugged terrain and still enjoy a cruise into the valley when you rejoin Peak to Creek.

122 Home Run ♦

Technically, this is only a "home run" if you live in one of the multimillion-dollar chalets in Kadenwood; in which case, you can ski to your doorstep. Dare to dream.

Local's Tip

We hope you all get a chance to ride Peak to Creek with five centimetres of fresh snow on top of perfect grooming. Once you have, you'll understand why this run became an instant classic and skiers scramble to be among the first to lay tracks on her in the morning! It's a truly incredible ride from the very summit of Whistler to the valley bottom, one you'll not soon forget. Watch the forecasts carefully and line up a perfect run!

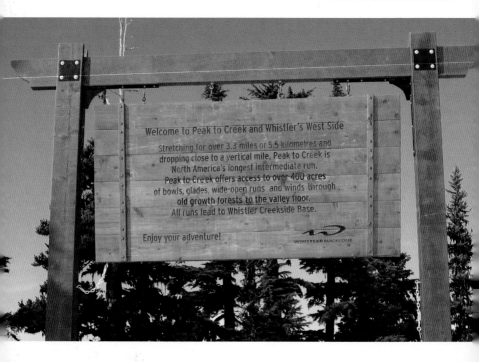

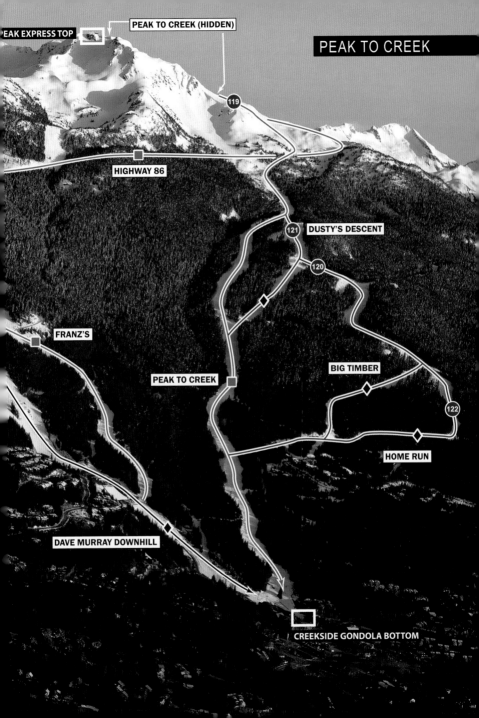

PEAK TO CREEK

EAK EXPRESS TOP   PEAK TO CREEK (HIDDEN)

119

HIGHWAY 86

121   DUSTY'S DESCENT

120

FRANZ'S

BIG TIMBER

PEAK TO CREEK

122

HOME RUN

DAVE MURRAY DOWNHILL

CREEKSIDE GONDOLA BOTTOM

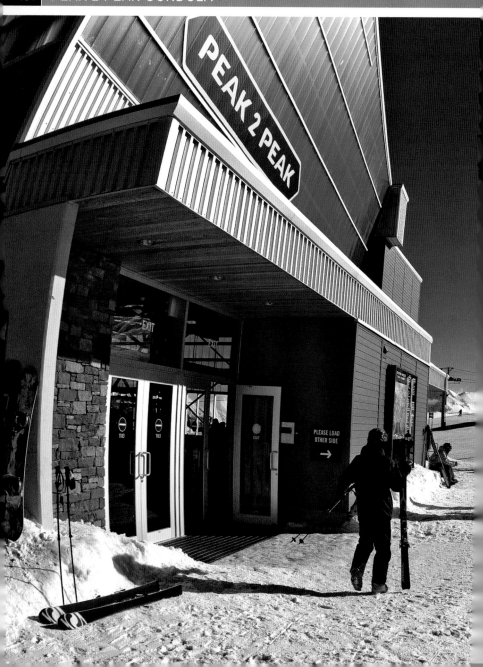

PEAK 2 PEAK GONDOLA

History and Construction

When Whistler Mountain merged with Blackcomb Skiing Enterprises in 1997, the idea of linking the two ski areas by an aerial tram was born. At first blush the idea sounded imposing. The steep-sided Fitzsimmons Creek valley that divides the two mountains is notorious for high winds, and the span in question would be over four kilometres long. Making the crossing would require a feat of engineering if it were possible at all. So, a few years later Whistler Blackcomb tasked Swiss-Austrian lift manufacturer Doppelmayr Garaventa with proposing a system that would effectively achieve the goal given the predominant conditions. The engineers came back with the plan to install two track cables across the span in

(continued on next page)

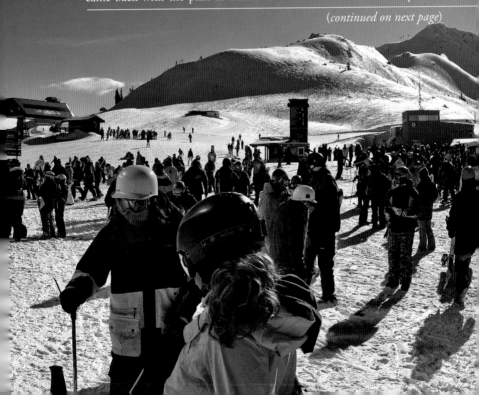

Statistics

Length: 4.4 kilometres
Number of Cabins: 28
Capacity: 4,100 people per hour
Line Speed: 7.5 metres per second
Ride Time: 11 minutes
Cost: $51 million Canadian

each direction, with one continuous haul rope in between. The idea was that the track cables would hold the gondola cabins steady against the wind (similar to outriggers supporting a canoe in rough seas), while the haul rope performed the heavy lifting, dragging the cabins across the valley. The system would require the installation of only four support towers and would be relatively low impact on the environment because no new roads would have to be built during the construction phase.

The idea made sense, and on May 21, 2007, Whistler Blackcomb officially broke ground on the Peak 2 Peak Gondola project. The work continued throughout the summer and into October, when the onset of winter conditions forced the project to go into a holding pattern. While snow blanketed the job site on the mountains, construction of the cabins, cables and machinery was fastidiously taking place in Europe. As soon as the snow melted, the work on the ground ramped back up. Throughout the summer of 2008, the two terminals were completed, the four towers were finished, and the cables were transported up the access road on Blackcomb. From this point, the project flew toward completion. The cables were winched into position and the two ends of the haul rope were spliced together to form a continuous loop. Twelve gondola cabins were placed onto the cables and on Sept. 19 the first cabins made the crossing from Whistler to Blackcomb. Weeks of extensive testing and certification lead way to the official opening of the Peak 2 Peak Gondola on December 12, 2008. The gondola currently holds world records for the longest unsupported span between ropeway towers (3.03 kilometres between towers 2 and 3) and the highest distance above the ground (436 metres).

Using the Peak 2 Peak Gondola

In 2005, the announcement that Whistler Blackcomb intended to place a gondola between the two mountains created a broad range of reactions. Citing the fact that the lift wouldn't open any new terrain, some local hardcores speculated that the lift would serve no purpose within the flow of their ski day. They forecast that the gondola would be nothing but a tourist attraction that would force the cost of season passes to rise. Some went even went as far as to swear they would never ride the lift as some sort of silent protest against further development.

Soon after opening, however, it became apparent that the Peak 2 Peak did, in fact, enhance the experience of the expert skier. Case in point, the gondola enables a capable expert to ski all of the alpine bowls on both mountains in one day. This would have required a descent into the valley along with a time-consuming lift ride back into the alpine in the days prior to the Peak 2 Peak. The gondola is also very useful when a setback in avalanche control delays the opening of the alpine area of one of the two mountains. The Peak 2 Peak offers a quick solution for switching sides, meaning that skiers are not as committed to one mountain or the other. Every powder day involves a bit of a gamble: Do you commit to Whistler or Blackcomb? Are you better off waiting for the Peak or Harmony, Glacier Express or 7th Heaven? The Peak 2 Peak can reduce the commitment factor by enabling a quick change if you alter your plans.

During the spring season, when the mountains periodically experience the debilitating phenomenon of mid-mountain fog, the Peak 2 Peak offers a quick escape to other zones less-affected due to sun exposure or prevailing winds. A simple glance across the valley may give you all the weather report you need, and the ride over will have you back in the sun in no time. The lift has also provided the ability to follow the light. Skiing and riding in flat light means the loss of ability to see contour and texture on the snow, effectively losing depth perception. Flat light occurs during overcast, cloudy conditions and when the mountain falls into the shade of its own shadow. The Peak 2 Peak allows you to ride in the early sun on Whistler's east-facing slopes and then switch over to Blackcomb for afternoon light on the west aspect. A final positive result of the lift are two new ski runs down the upper sections of the lift line. Zudrell's Run (Whistler) and Luger's Run (Blackcomb) are both described within this book.

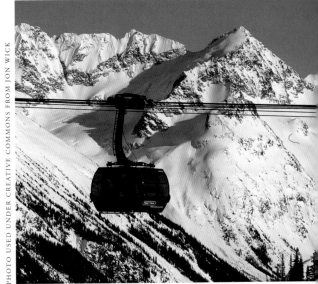

PHOTO USED UNDER CREATIVE COMMONS FROM JON WICK

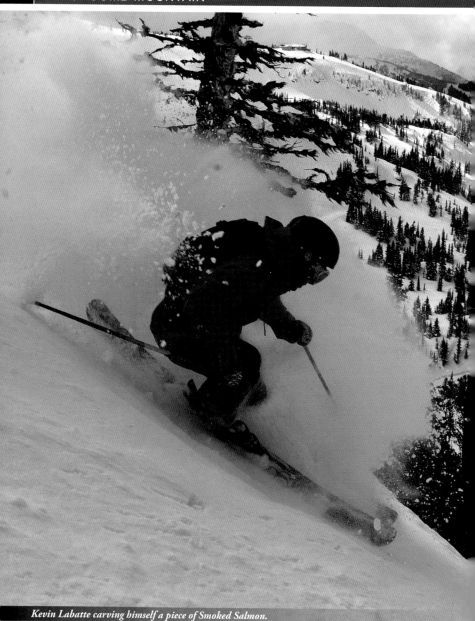

Kevin Labatte carving himself a piece of Smoked Salmon.

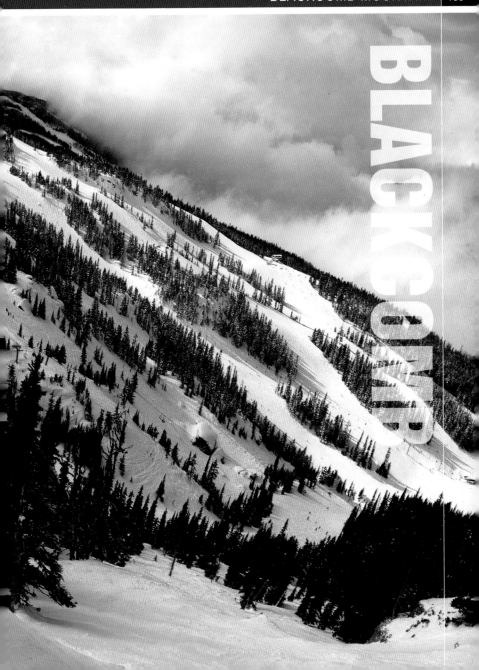

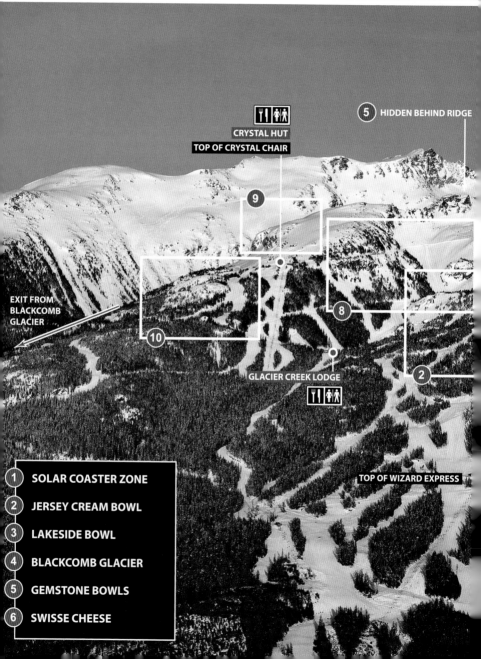

CRYSTAL HUT
TOP OF CRYSTAL CHAIR

(5) HIDDEN BEHIND RIDGE

9

EXIT FROM
BLACKCOMB
GLACIER

8

10

GLACIER CREEK LODGE

2

TOP OF WIZARD EXPRESS

1 **SOLAR COASTER ZONE**

2 **JERSEY CREAM BOWL**

3 **LAKESIDE BOWL**

4 **BLACKCOMB GLACIER**

5 **GEMSTONE BOWLS**

6 **SWISSE CHEESE**

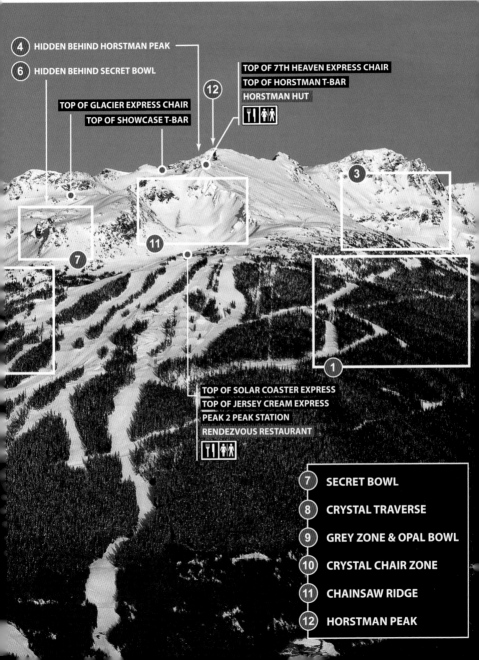

4 HIDDEN BEHIND HORSTMAN PEAK

6 HIDDEN BEHIND SECRET BOWL

TOP OF 7TH HEAVEN EXPRESS CHAIR
TOP OF HORSTMAN T-BAR
HORSTMAN HUT

12

TOP OF GLACIER EXPRESS CHAIR
TOP OF SHOWCASE T-BAR

3

11

7

1

TOP OF SOLAR COASTER EXPRESS
TOP OF JERSEY CREAM EXPRESS
PEAK 2 PEAK STATION
RENDEZVOUS RESTAURANT

7 SECRET BOWL

8 CRYSTAL TRAVERSE

9 GREY ZONE & OPAL BOWL

10 CRYSTAL CHAIR ZONE

11 CHAINSAW RIDGE

12 HORSTMAN PEAK

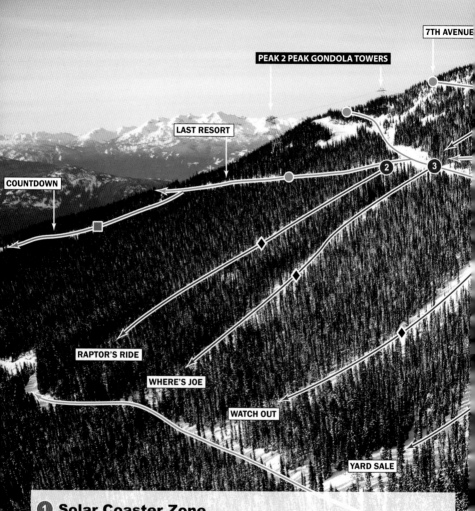

7TH AVENUE

PEAK 2 PEAK GONDOLA TOWERS

LAST RESORT

COUNTDOWN

2

3

RAPTOR'S RIDE

WHERE'S JOE

WATCH OUT

YARD SALE

① Solar Coaster Zone

Even in the most heinous storms, when the high alpine remains closed, there is lots of terrain in the sub-alpine on Blackcomb that beats sitting at home with your iPad. Check these out:

① Lines off 7th Avenue ♦ ★★

There are some short, steep lines that drop off 7th Avenue through tight trees to Express Way below.

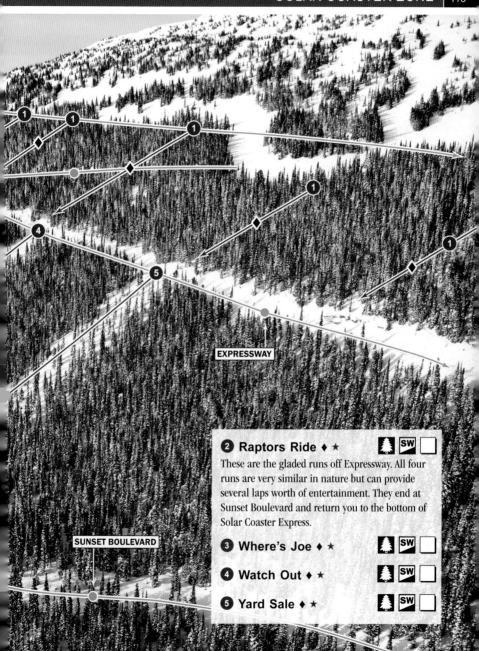

EXPRESSWAY

SUNSET BOULEVARD

② Raptors Ride ♦ ★

These are the gladed runs off Expressway. All four runs are very similar in nature but can provide several laps worth of entertainment. They end at Sunset Boulevard and return you to the bottom of Solar Coaster Express.

③ Where's Joe ♦ ★

④ Watch Out ♦ ★

⑤ Yard Sale ♦ ★

❻ Renegade Glade ♦ ★★

Renegade Glade and Little cub are two often neglected glade runs found off Last Resort. The patrol loves these runs because they sometimes have untouched powder left at the end of the day for sweep!

❼ Little Cub ♦ ★★

❽ Luger's Run ♦ ★

The Peak 2 Peak lift line. Named after Peter Luger, the head engineer for Doppelmayr Garaventa, the Swiss-Austrian company responsible for designing and installing the gondola. The run ends at Sunset Boulevard, which can be ridden back to the Solar Coaster Express.

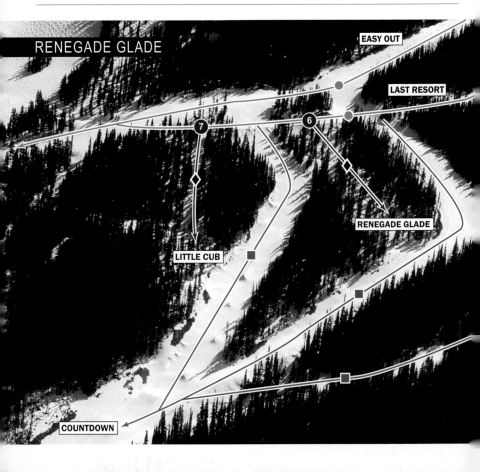

RENEGADE GLADE

EASY OUT

LAST RESORT

RENEGADE GLADE

LITTLE CUB

COUNTDOWN

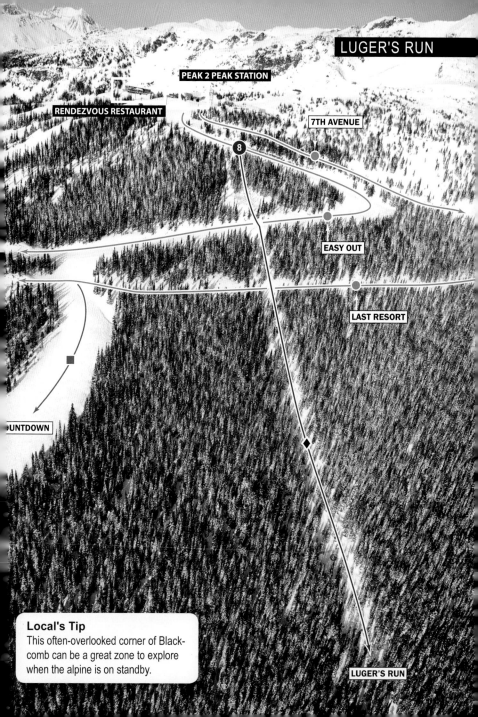

LUGER'S RUN

PEAK 2 PEAK STATION

RENDEZVOUS RESTAURANT

7TH AVENUE

8

EASY OUT

LAST RESORT

UNTDOWN

Local's Tip
This often-overlooked corner of Black-comb can be a great zone to explore when the alpine is on standby.

LUGER'S RUN

② Jersey Cream Bowl

This sub-alpine area is usually one of the first zones to get avalanche clearance. It can be opened even if there is active avalanche control being conducted on the alpine slopes above. This area has some short but fun chutes, small drops, and a traverse out to some good glades and steeps.

❾ Hot Tub ♦ ★

Short little convex slope off the top of the Jersey Cream Express chair. Named after the round hot-tub-looking water tower.

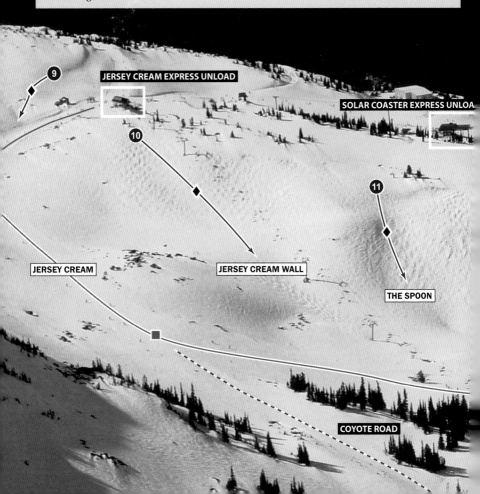

⑩ Jersey Cream Wall ♦

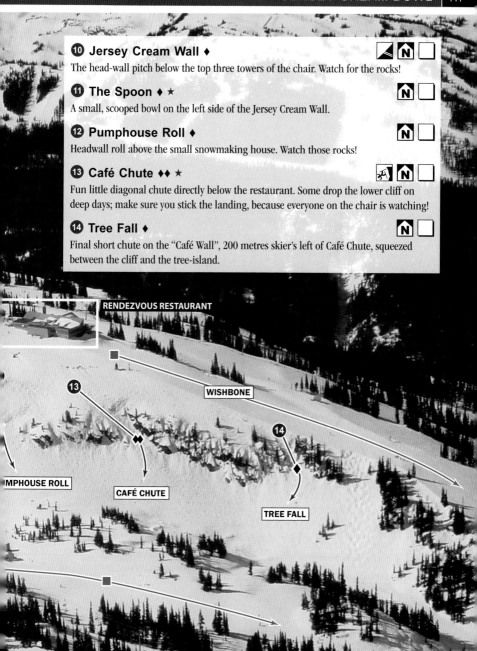

The head-wall pitch below the top three towers of the chair. Watch for the rocks!

⑪ The Spoon ♦ ★

A small, scooped bowl on the left side of the Jersey Cream Wall.

⑫ Pumphouse Roll ♦

Headwall roll above the small snowmaking house. Watch those rocks!

⑬ Café Chute ♦♦ ★

Fun little diagonal chute directly below the restaurant. Some drop the lower cliff on deep days; make sure you stick the landing, because everyone on the chair is watching!

⑭ Tree Fall ♦

Final short chute on the "Café Wall", 200 metres skier's left of Café Chute, squeezed between the cliff and the tree-island.

RENDEZVOUS RESTAURANT

⑬ WISHBONE

⑭

IMPHOUSE ROLL

CAFÉ CHUTE

TREE FALL

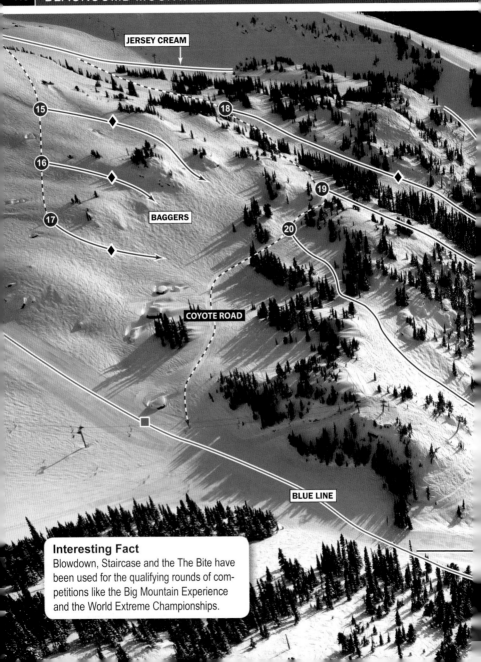

JERSEY CREAM

15

18

16

17

BAGGERS

19

20

COYOTE ROAD

BLUE LINE

Interesting Fact
Blowdown, Staircase and the The Bite have
been used for the qualifying rounds of competitions like the Big Mountain Experience
and the World Extreme Championships.

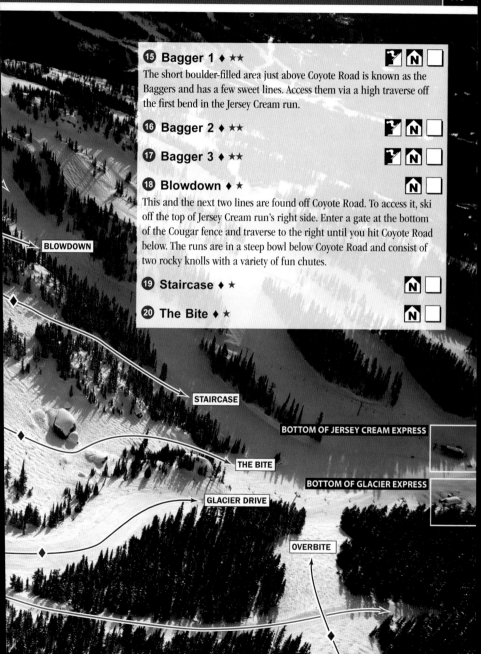

⑮ Bagger 1 ♦ ★★

The short boulder-filled area just above Coyote Road is known as the Baggers and has a few sweet lines. Access them via a high traverse off the first bend in the Jersey Cream run.

⑯ Bagger 2 ♦ ★★

⑰ Bagger 3 ♦ ★★

⑱ Blowdown ♦ ★

This and the next two lines are found off Coyote Road. To access it, ski off the top of Jersey Cream run's right side. Enter a gate at the bottom of the Cougar fence and traverse to the right until you hit Coyote Road below. The runs are in a steep bowl below Coyote Road and consist of two rocky knolls with a variety of fun chutes.

⑲ Staircase ♦ ★

⑳ The Bite ♦ ★

BLOWDOWN

STAIRCASE

BOTTOM OF JERSEY CREAM EXPRESS

THE BITE

BOTTOM OF GLACIER EXPRESS

GLACIER DRIVE

OVERBITE

③ **Lakeside Bowl**

This is the massive bowl visible as you ride up the 7th Heaven chair. Get off at the top and head right along Green Line to the first corner. Continue traversing to the fence line and enter a gate to Lakeside Bowl. The traverse is serious and can be more hazardous than any of the actual skiing!

㉑ **Traverse Pillow** ♦ ★

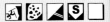

Once you enter through the gate and take the high traverse toward the bowl, you reach a point where you can sidestep up under a ski patrol bomb tram. This slope is called the Pillow, and when skied from below the cliffs, it makes for quick access to good powder.

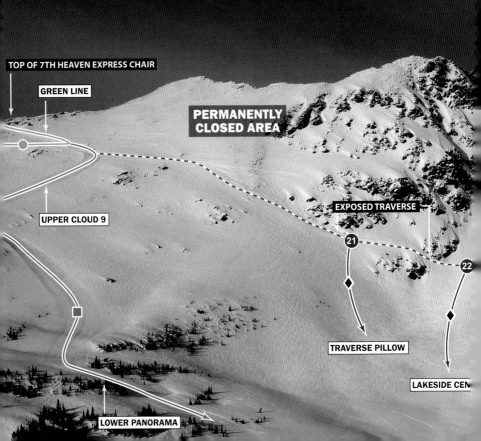

TOP OF 7TH HEAVEN EXPRESS CHAIR

GREEN LINE

PERMANENTLY CLOSED AREA

UPPER CLOUD 9

EXPOSED TRAVERSE

㉑

㉒

TRAVERSE PILLOW

LAKESIDE CEN

LOWER PANORAMA

㉒ Lakeside Centre ♦ ★★★

  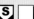

Traverse to the centre of the massive bowl and rip it up! Don't even think of hiking above the traverse. It's a permanent closure and you'll lose your pass!

㉓ Heartthrob ♦ ★★

This is the small rock outcrop mid-bowl. Ski across the top and shred the left side.

㉔ I.D. Low ♦♦ ★★

Continue the rising traverse, stepping up over a lateral cornice. Ski back in and air if you dare!

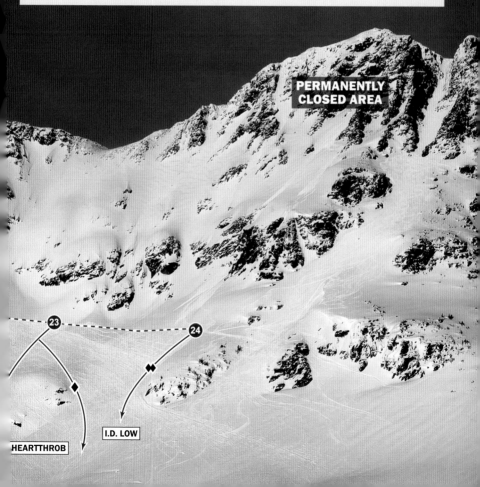

PERMANENTLY CLOSED AREA

I.D. LOW

HEARTTHROB

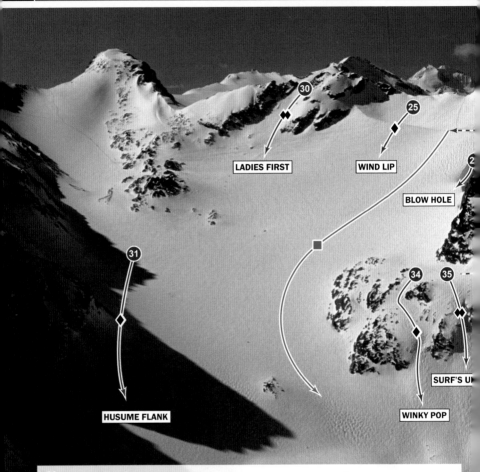

LADIES FIRST

WIND LIP

BLOW HOLE

HUSUME FLANK

WINKY POP

SURF'S U

④ Blackcomb Glacier

As the highest lift on the mountain, Showcase T-Bar accesses the Blackcomb Glacier and the world-famous Wind Lip. In major storms, this lift will stay closed in order to keep people out of the massive terrain behind the ridge, which often experiences avalanches up to Class 4 in size!

㉕ The Wind Lip ♦ ★

The Wind Lip is a giant snow moat created by the force of the wind that comes over the ridge. This, combined with the steep slope below, makes it the best natural booter in the world! Made famous in countless ski and snowboard movies, this is a must-do for any would-be huckster.

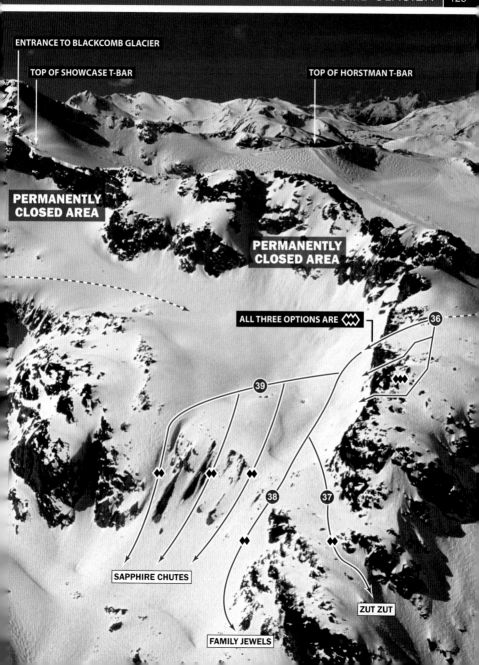

ENTRANCE TO BLACKCOMB GLACIER

TOP OF SHOWCASE T-BAR

TOP OF HORSTMAN T-BAR

PERMANENTLY CLOSED AREA

PERMANENTLY CLOSED AREA

ALL THREE OPTIONS ARE

36

39

38

37

SAPPHIRE CHUTES

ZUT ZUT

FAMILY JEWELS

26 The Blowhole ♦♦ ★★★

Get off the Showcase T-Bar and traverse right for 50 metres to a boot-pack up to the Blackcomb Glacier gate. Once through, this huge feature is on your left. To capture the glory, have your photographer shoot from the ridge behind the wooden sign or from the bottom, looking up.

27 Java ♦ ★

Hike along the Wind Lip and climb to the ridge. Traverse around the rocks and up to a chute. Ski back into the glacier watching out for crevasses.

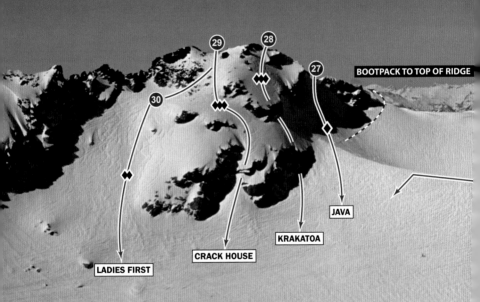

BOOTPACK TO TOP OF RIDGE

JAVA

KRAKATOA

CRACK HOUSE

LADIES FIRST

Interesting Fact

Ladies First is named in honour of Whistler patroller, Cathy Jewett, who was the first to "ski" the line back in 1984. On that fateful day, Jewett dropped in and instantly set off an avalanche that she rode down the slope until she was able to self-arrest with her gloved fingers. "The sad thing is that I really didn't ski it that day!" said Jewett, years later.

28 Krakatoa ◆◆◆ ★★

Access as above. Hike around the back of the rock ridge to the top. Serious cornice hazard exists! This run involves drops over two rock bands that can be anywhere from 2–10 metres (6–30 feet) depending on the snow cover.

29 Crack House ◆◆◆ ★

Hike to the top as for Ladies First. Negotiate around the upper cliff to the chute with mandatory air.

© SCOTT FLAVELLE

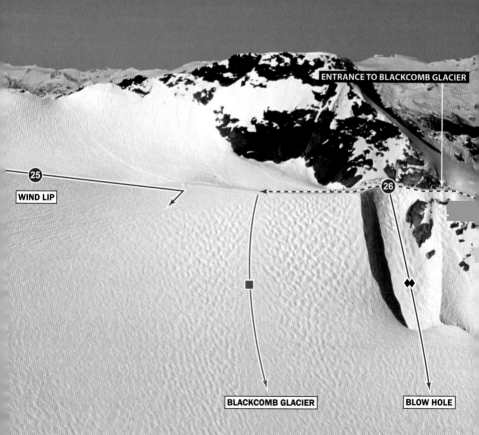

ENTRANCE TO BLACKCOMB GLACIER

25

WIND LIP

26

BLACKCOMB GLACIER

BLOW HOLE

30 Ladies First ♦♦ ★★★

Continue along the rock ridge—past the notch, over the top, and in near the Permanent Closure fence that is placed here to keep skiers out of Upper Lakeside Bowl. Sometimes, you have to carry your boards down and right, over some rocks.

31 Husume Flank ♦ ★★

Great link up with Ladies First. Traverse to the right side of Blackcomb Glacier. This run is inside the ski area but close to the boundary line, which should be designated with signs. Some seriously deep turns can be had here when the prevailing winds work to deposit light snow in the fan.

Local's Tip
The broad, unlabeled chute in the picture on page 127 is called Husume. It is outside of the ski area boundary and does not receive regular avalanche control. If you want to sample it, hire a local guide to take you in there. It's a backcountry classic.

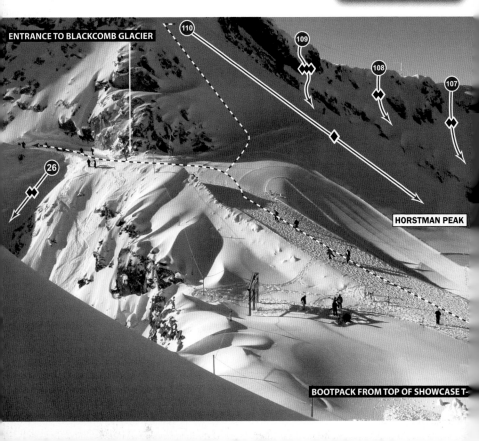

ENTRANCE TO BLACKCOMB GLACIER

110

109

108

107

26

HORSTMAN PEAK

BOOTPACK FROM TOP OF SHOWCASE T-

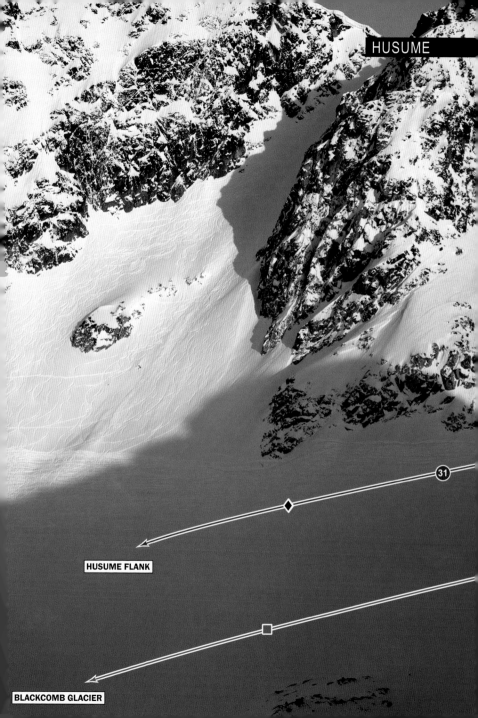

HUSUME

31

HUSUME FLANK

BLACKCOMB GLACIER

⑤ Gemstone Bowls

The Glacier Express chairlift takes you from the Jersey Cream Flats (outside of the Glacier Creek mega-restaurant) up to the bottom of Horstman Glacier and the two T-bars. "G.E." is the gateway to Spanky's Ladder bootpack and the Gemstone Bowls of Garnet, Ruby, Diamond, and Sapphire. In some storms, this lift provides the highest access on the mountain and Spanky's Ladder may remain closed. If this is the case, don't worry, there's still plenty of high-alpine terrain in the Cougar and Secret areas!

㉜ Spanky's Ladder

No easy way out from here! Spanky's Ladder is the 15-metre bootpack that you must hike up to access the ridge between Crystal Traverse and the Blackcomb Glacier valley. Get off Glacier Express and turn left, traverse below the ridge for 400 metres to the bottom of a steep snow slope. From here, hike up and through the gate.

TRAVERSE TO CHIMNEY BOOTPACK, ACCESS TO GREY ZONE AND OPAL BOWL

CRYSTAL TRAVERSE

BOTTOM OF HORSTMAN T-BAR

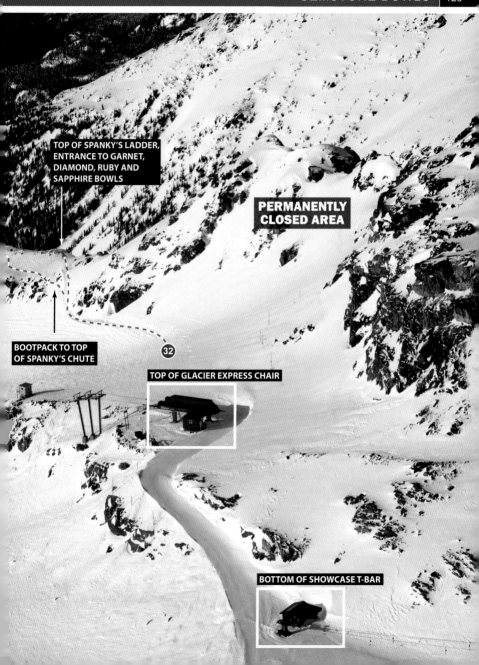

TOP OF SPANKY'S LADDER, ENTRANCE TO GARNET, DIAMOND, RUBY AND SAPPHIRE BOWLS

PERMANENTLY CLOSED AREA

BOOTPACK TO TOP OF SPANKY'S CHUTE

32

TOP OF GLACIER EXPRESS CHAIR

BOTTOM OF SHOWCASE T-BAR

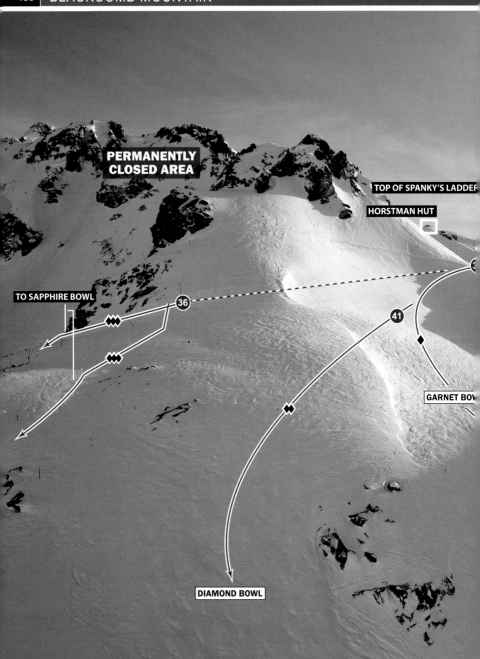

PERMANENTLY CLOSED AREA

TOP OF SPANKY'S LADDER

HORSTMAN HUT

TO SAPPHIRE BOWL

36

41

GARNET BOWL

DIAMOND BOWL

33 Garnet Bowl ♦ ★

Garnet is the upper basin that funnels you into Sapphire, Diamond, and Ruby Bowls. From the gate at the top of Spanky's Ladder, a traverse to the right leads to Sapphire Bowl, to the left leads to Ruby, and if you go straight, you end up in Diamond bowl.

Local's Tip
Of all the choices the Gemstone Bowls have to offer, a run down Diamond Bowl offers the most vertical with the least amount of traversing. Enjoy!

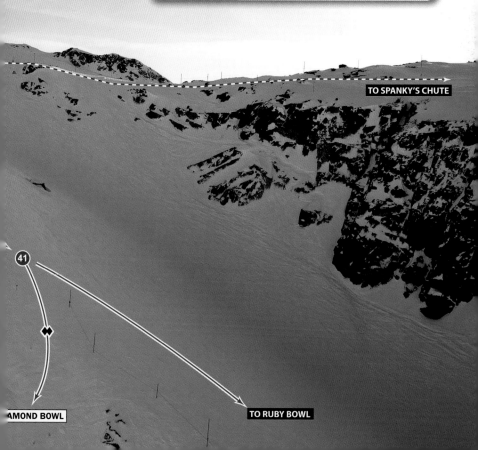

TO SPANKY'S CHUTE

41

◆◆

AMOND BOWL

TO RUBY BOWL

34 Winky Pop ♦ ★★

Traverse left through the labyrinth of rocks on the wide bench below the Blowhole.

35 Surf's Up ♦♦ ★★★

Access is the same as for Winky Pop, only sidestep up a further 10 to 15 metres to gain the chute at the top of Surf's Up.

36 Sapphire Bowl ♦♦♦ ★★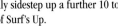

The toughest of the bowls to get into, Sapphire requires a tricky bit of navigation through rocks on the edge of a cliff. Traverse right in Garnet Bowl to a bench that splits into an upper and lower traverse line. Take the lower line and sketch your way into the Bowl.

37 Zut Zut ♦♦ ★★★

A good way to get to Diamond from Sapphire Bowl, this line forms a fat cornice and snow loads so deeply in here you may need a snorkel!

38 Family Jewels ♦♦ ★★

The skier's left-most line through Sapphire Bowl eventually traverses left on a bench into Diamond Bowl.

39 Sapphire Chutes ♦♦ ★★★

The upper bowl divides into three chutes lower down through old lateral moraines.

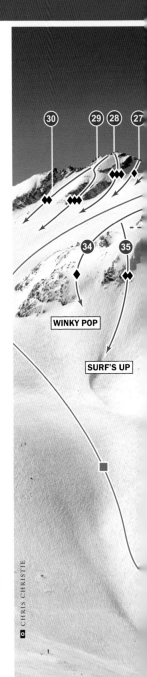

WINKY POP

SURF'S UP

> **Interesting Fact**
> Unfortunately, Blackcomb Glacier is experiencing an annual recession of between five and ten metres. By the year 2050, it will likely become a casualty of our changing climate.

© CHRIS CHRISTIE

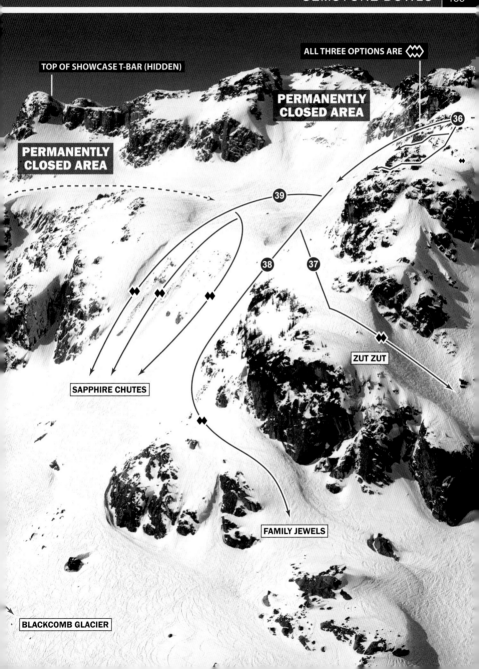

TOP OF SHOWCASE T-BAR (HIDDEN)

ALL THREE OPTIONS ARE

PERMANENTLY CLOSED AREA

PERMANENTLY CLOSED AREA

36

39

38 37

SAPPHIRE CHUTES

ZUT ZUT

FAMILY JEWELS

BLACKCOMB GLACIER

40 Wild Thing ♦♦ ★★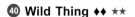

Another way into Diamond, on the shoulder from Sapphire Bowl

41 Diamond Bowl ♦♦ ★★★

Diamond has three entrances from Garnet: Diamond Roll (right), Diamond Centre, and Diamond Left.

42 Calvin ♦♦ ★★

Enter via Diamond Left and hook left after the diagonal ramp to the slope below the big cliff. Look up and wonder what the guy who tried to jump into this slope from above was thinking!

43 Hobbes ♦♦ ★★

Directly below Calvin are some short chutes divided by rock bluffs. Hobbes offers many variations, most of which are good.

44 Bad Attitude ♦♦♦ ★★★

"B.A." is accessed by a traverse left from Calvin through some exposed terrain.

45 Mid-Bowl Roll/Gully ♦♦ ★★

In the centre of Diamond Bowl, you have a choice between Mid-bowl Roll (right), and Mid-bowl Gully (left).

Local's Tip

The steepness and true north aspect of Zut Zut aid in the preservation of snow quality on the slope. If the sun has torched the neighboring lines, this might be your best bet.

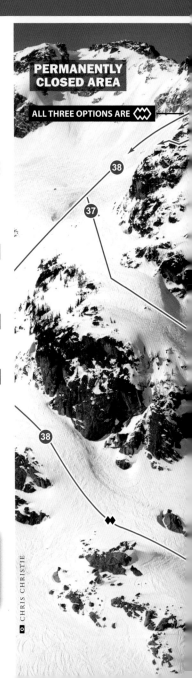

PERMANENTLY CLOSED AREA

ALL THREE OPTIONS ARE

38

37

38

CHRIS CHRISTIE

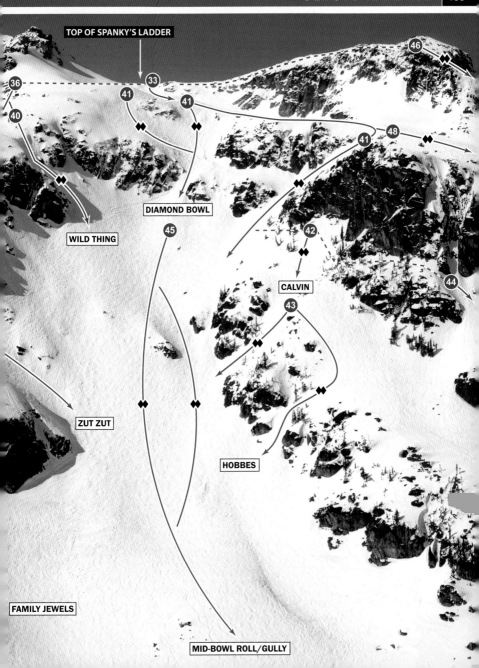

TOP OF SPANKY'S LADDER

36

40

33

41

41

46

48

41

DIAMOND BOWL

WILD THING

45

42

CALVIN

44

43

ZUT ZUT

HOBBES

FAMILY JEWELS

MID-BOWL ROLL/GULLY

46 Spanky's Chute ♦♦ ★★★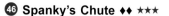

From the top of Spanky's Ladder, stay on the ridge and traverse left along the fence until you can slide into the steep chute. Several variations are possible to get into the bowl.

47 Gummy Bear ♦♦ ★★★

A great pocket snowfield accessed high via Spanky's Chute or low via Spanky's Shoulder.

48 Spanky's Shoulder ♦♦ ★★★

From the top of the Ladder, drop into Garnet Bowl and traverse left below the cliffs. You will arrive at the mellower, convex slope that rolls into Ruby Bowl.

49 Skid Lips ♦♦ ★★

From the Spanky's Shoulder entrance, drop down the ridge to the edge of the cliff and shred the line on the tight skier's right through the rocks.

50 Playland ♦♦ ★★★

From the bottom of Skid Lips, tuck right, under the cliff. Traverse right, into the super-fun gully. Enjoy! It is called Playland for a reason!

51 Shredder ♦♦ ★★

Traverse the upper bowl from Spanky's Chute to the far skier's left. The tight couloir above is called Shredder. Slide in the bottom and rip it until your legs burn.

52 Midway Rock ♦♦ ★

Midway refers to the cliff in the upper third of the Bowl. There are two lines, Midway Left and Midway Right. Both are good.

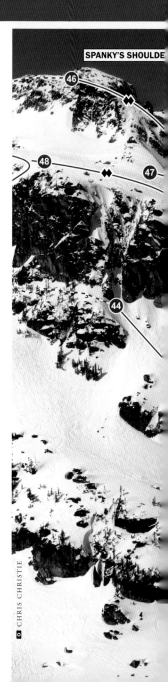

SPANKY'S SHOULDE

46

48

47

44

© CHRIS CHRISTIE

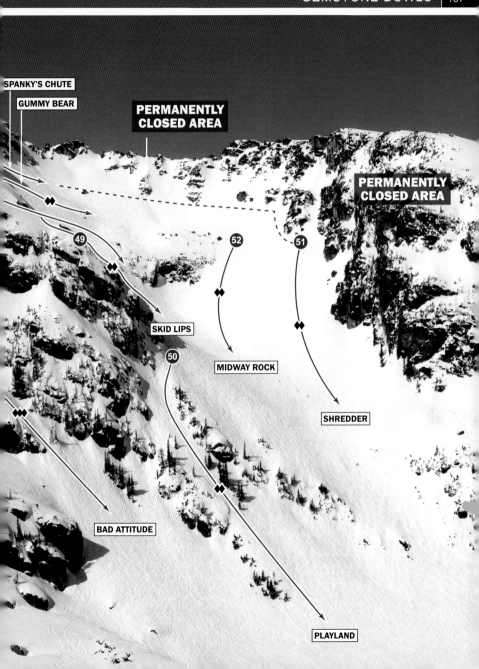

SPANKY'S CHUTE

GUMMY BEAR

PERMANENTLY CLOSED AREA

PERMANENTLY CLOSED AREA

49

52

51

SKID LIPS

MIDWAY ROCK

SHREDDER

50

BAD ATTITUDE

PLAYLAND

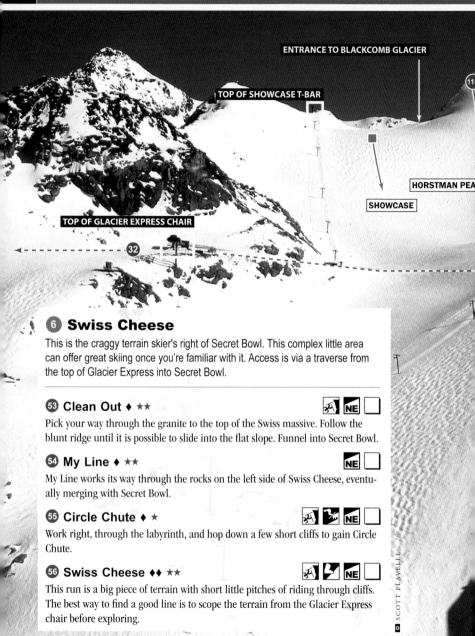

ENTRANCE TO BLACKCOMB GLACIER

110

TOP OF SHOWCASE T-BAR

HORSTMAN PEA

SHOWCASE

TOP OF GLACIER EXPRESS CHAIR

32

© SCOTT FLAVELLE

6 Swiss Cheese

This is the craggy terrain skier's right of Secret Bowl. This complex little area can offer great skiing once you're familiar with it. Access is via a traverse from the top of Glacier Express into Secret Bowl.

53 Clean Out ♦ ★★

Pick your way through the granite to the top of the Swiss massive. Follow the blunt ridge until it is possible to slide into the flat slope. Funnel into Secret Bowl.

54 My Line ♦ ★★

My Line works its way through the rocks on the left side of Swiss Cheese, eventually merging with Secret Bowl.

55 Circle Chute ♦ ★

Work right, through the labyrinth, and hop down a few short cliffs to gain Circle Chute.

56 Swiss Cheese ♦♦ ★★

This run is a big piece of terrain with short little pitches of riding through cliffs. The best way to find a good line is to scope the terrain from the Glacier Express chair before exploring.

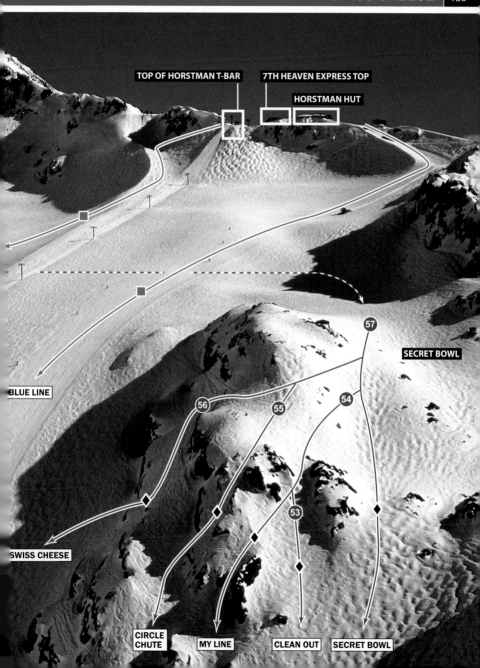

TOP OF HORSTMAN T-BAR

7TH HEAVEN EXPRESS TOP

HORSTMAN HUT

SECRET BOWL

57

BLUE LINE

56

55

54

53

SWISS CHEESE

CIRCLE CHUTE

MY LINE

CLEAN OUT

SECRET BOWL

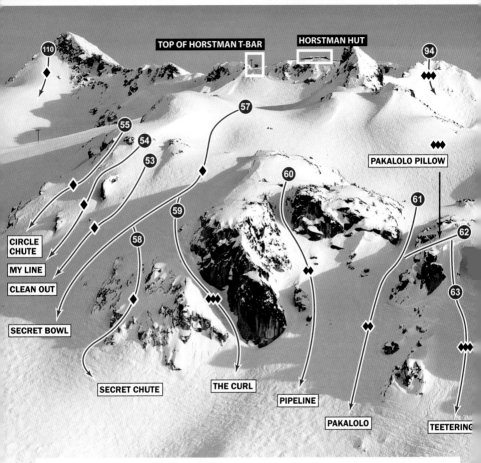

TOP OF HORSTMAN T-BAR

HORSTMAN HUT

110
94

57

55
54
53

PAKALOLO PILLOW

60

61

59
62

58

CIRCLE CHUTE

MY LINE

CLEAN OUT

63

SECRET BOWL

SECRET CHUTE

THE CURL

PIPELINE

PAKALOLO

TEETERING

7 Secret Bowl

Secret Bowl is perched between Blackcomb Bowl (Chainsaw Ridge) and the Glacier Express chairlift. Below the bowl are a number of excellent lines and chutes, all of which funnel down into the Jersey Cream bowl.

57 Secret Bowl ♦ ★★★

Follow the natural line into the col between the Swiss Cheese zone and Secret Basin.

58 Secret Chute ♦ ★★★

Ski the left side of Secret Bowl and watch for the chute that develops in the lower third of the bowl.

59 The Curl ♦♦♦ ★★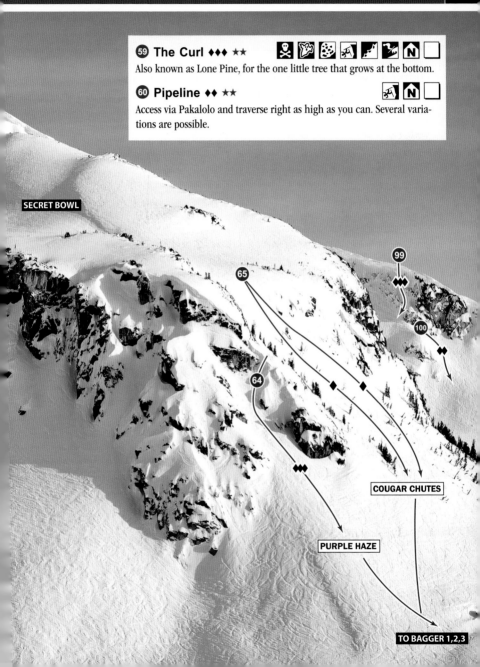
Also known as Lone Pine, for the one little tree that grows at the bottom.

60 Pipeline ♦♦ ★★
Access via Pakalolo and traverse right as high as you can. Several variations are possible.

SECRET BOWL

65

99

100

64

COUGAR CHUTES

PURPLE HAZE

TO BAGGER 1,2,3

61 Pakalolo ♦♦ ★★★

Traverse to Secret Basin, but stay left of the bowl and look for the obvious entrance into this classic couloir. Photo on page 140.

62 Pakalolo Pillow ♦♦♦ ★★★

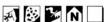

The burlier entrance into the couloir. Stay even farther left and work your way around the rocks to gain access to the edge of the drop in. Photo on page 140.

63 Teetering ♦♦♦ ★

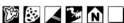

Named after the Wile E. Coyote rock perched on the edge of the cliff another 30 metres left, Teetering is the STEEP entrance into this chute. Access depends on snow coverage!

64 Purple Haze ♦♦♦ ★★

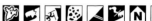

Purple Haze and Cougar Chutes, both visible from the top third of the Jersey Cream chair, are accessed via the Secret Basin and a continuous traverse left, past the sign line. To ski Purple Haze, enter the top of the Cougar Chute Right and traverse right, on the flat bench with the two small islands of trees. Creep to the edge below the cornice and scope it out! Don't miss your first turn, because you might not get a second one!

65 Cougar Chutes ♦♦ ★★

Several lines are possible through the chutes and boulders. Watch out for the pungy trees!

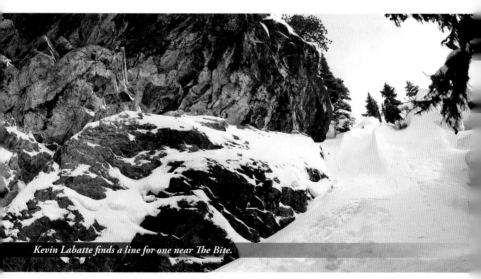

Kevin Labatte finds a line for one near The Bite.

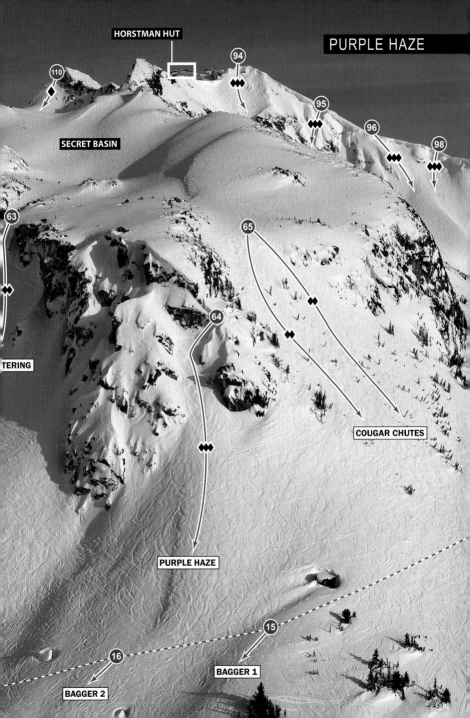

PURPLE HAZE

HORSTMAN HUT

SECRET BASIN

TERING

COUGAR CHUTES

PURPLE HAZE

BAGGER 1

BAGGER 2

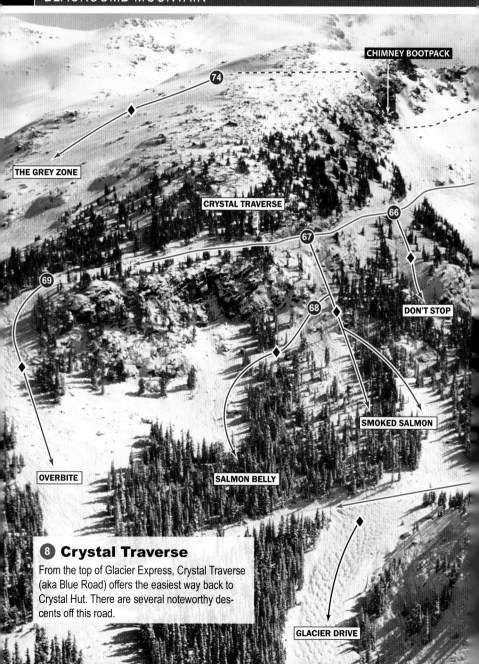

CHIMNEY BOOTPACK

74

THE GREY ZONE

CRYSTAL TRAVERSE

66

67

69

68

DON'T STOP

SMOKED SALMON

OVERBITE

SALMON BELLY

8 Crystal Traverse

From the top of Glacier Express, Crystal Traverse (aka Blue Road) offers the easiest way back to Crystal Hut. There are several noteworthy descents off this road.

GLACIER DRIVE

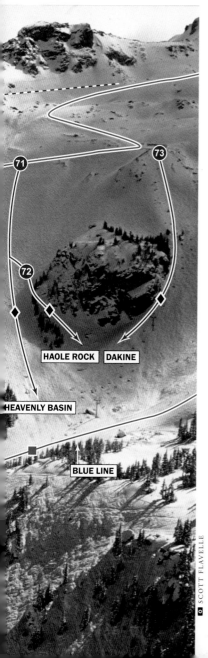

66 Don't Stop ◆ ★★★

Past Heavenly Basin, there are three great lines off Crystal Road, before you reach the Crystal Hut restaurant. First comes Don't Stop, the cool S-shaped chute through the trees.

67 Smoked Salmon ◆ ★★★

The second chute through the trees and the most sustained of the three. There are some boulders in this zone that make great natural hucks.

68 Salmon Belly ◆ ★★

The third route, closest to the Hot Rocks cliff face, the Belly widens out below the cliff and has room for more fresh lines.

69 Overbite ◆ ★

This cut run is chronically rocky and is best avoided unless it's a 30-centimetre-plus day!

70 Davies Dervish ◆ ★★

(No photo - see mountain map) This bumpy horror show is the site of World Cup mogul events. Call your physiotherapist for an appointment before you drop in! Still interested? Access is off Blue Line beyond Overbite.

71 Heavenly Basin ◆ ★★

Find it just off the Crystal Road, past the hairpin turn. Large variation in aspect ensures quality snow.

72 Haole Rock ◆ ★

Skier's left in Heavenly Basin. The big rock outcrop is Haole Rock. This line is funky terrain between the thin trees and the rock.

73 Dakine ◆ ★★

This refers to the line skier's left of the huge Haole rock, under the chair. This run can fetch epic snow. If you hit it first make it look good!

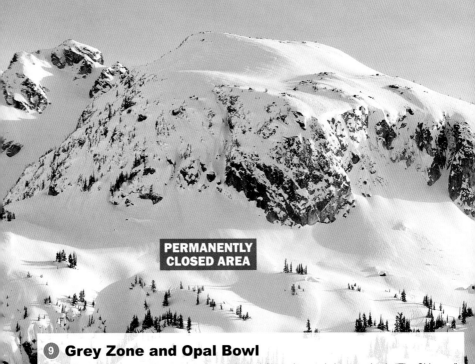

PERMANENTLY
CLOSED AREA

9 Grey Zone and Opal Bowl

This high-alpine ridge and bowl sit above the Crystal Chair. Access is best made via "The Chimney" (page 142), a bootpack above the Crystal Traverse. To find it, follow the Crystal Traverse from the top of Glacier Express for 1,200 metres, until the sharp left corner. Leave the road and traverse the boulder-strewn upper Heavenly Basin to the short hike below the cliffs at the first tree island.

74 The Grey Zone ◆ ★

From the top of The Chimney, descend this wide ridge to the Crystal Hut. Great lower-angle powder skiing. Watch for boulders!

75 Molly's Reach ◆◆ ★

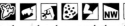

Cross the Grey Zone to the fence on skier's right. Follow the fence to the end and approach the edge carefully to find a way in.

76 Danger Bay ◆◆ ★★

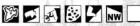

Same as Molly's, only traverse the ridge farther and find your way into the chute from right to left.

77 Front Page Challenge ♦ ★★★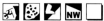

The lowest and easiest way into the Opal Bowl before you reach the traverse in from Crystal Chair. Take this line first and scope out the others.

78 Romper Room ♦ ★★

Traverse across Opal Bowl toward the trees. When you hit the boundary disks, turn down and shred the fun rolling terrain. Traverse left after 200 metres, to get back to Ridge Runner.

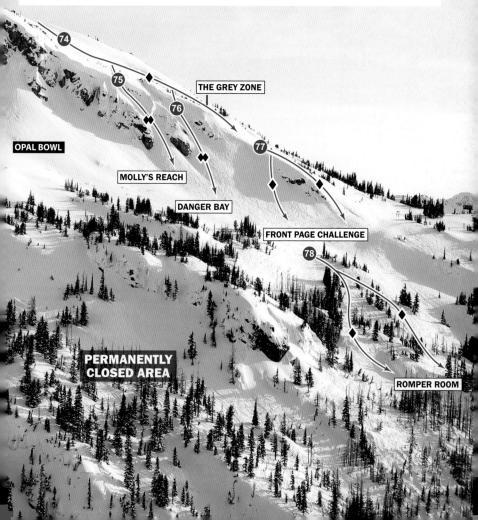

THE GREY ZONE

OPAL BOWL

MOLLY'S REACH

DANGER BAY

FRONT PAGE CHALLENGE

PERMANENTLY CLOSED AREA

ROMPER ROOM

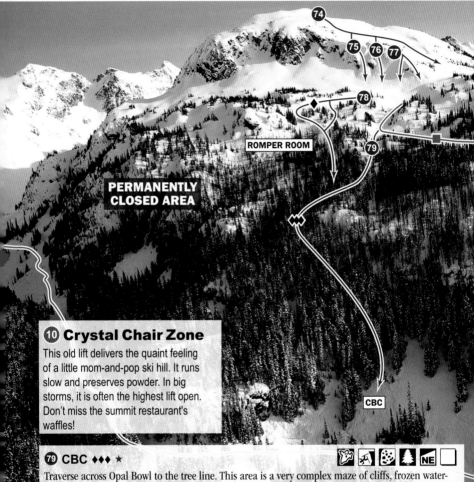

74

75 76 77

78

ROMPER ROOM

79

PERMANENTLY
CLOSED AREA

CBC

10 Crystal Chair Zone

This old lift delivers the quaint feeling of a little mom-and-pop ski hill. It runs slow and preserves powder. In big storms, it is often the highest lift open. Don't miss the summit restaurant's waffles!

79 CBC ♦♦♦ ★

Traverse across Opal Bowl to the tree line. This area is a very complex maze of cliffs, frozen waterfalls, and chutes. Don't go in there without a knowledgeable guide!

80 Outer Limits ♦♦ ★

Outer Limits can be either heaven or hell depending on the snow! Access is through the big wooden gate on the skier's right of Ridge Runner.

81 Arthur's Choice ♦ ★

This and the next two gladed runs are the same as Outer Limits, but less steep. All are definitely worth a look when the snow is good.

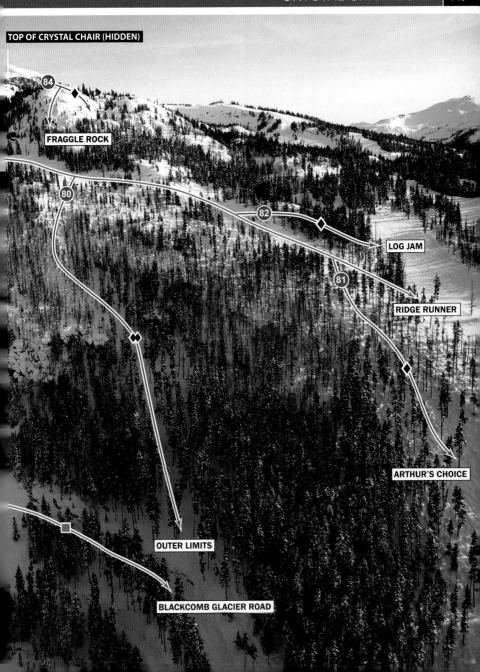

TOP OF CRYSTAL CHAIR (HIDDEN)

FRAGGLE ROCK

LOG JAM

RIDGE RUNNER

ARTHUR'S CHOICE

OUTER LIMITS

BLACKCOMB GLACIER ROAD

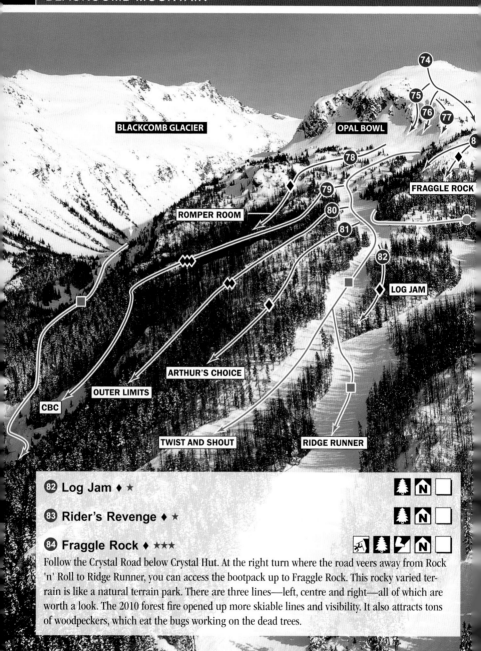

BLACKCOMB GLACIER

OPAL BOWL

FRAGGLE ROCK

ROMPER ROOM

LOG JAM

ARTHUR'S CHOICE

OUTER LIMITS

CBC

TWIST AND SHOUT

RIDGE RUNNER

82 Log Jam ♦ ★

83 Rider's Revenge ♦ ★

84 Fraggle Rock ♦ ★★★

Follow the Crystal Road below Crystal Hut. At the right turn where the road veers away from Rock 'n' Roll to Ridge Runner, you can access the bootpack up to Fraggle Rock. This rocky varied terrain is like a natural terrain park. There are three lines—left, centre and right—all of which are worth a look. The 2010 forest fire opened up more skiable lines and visibility. It also attracts tons of woodpeckers, which eat the bugs working on the dead trees.

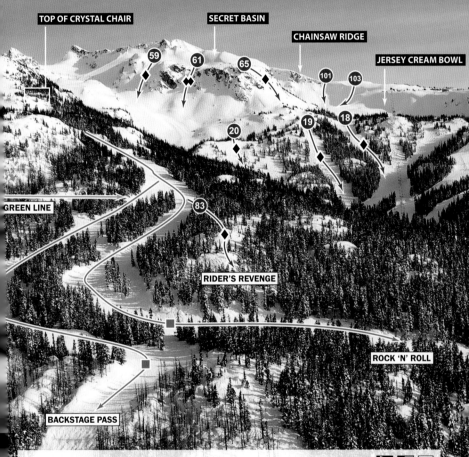

TOP OF CRYSTAL CHAIR

SECRET BASIN

CHAINSAW RIDGE

JERSEY CREAM BOWL

59

61

65

101

103

19

18

20

GREEN LINE

83

RIDER'S REVENGE

ROCK 'N' ROLL

BACKSTAGE PASS

85 Crystal Glide Cliffs ♦♦ ★★

(No photo) At the bottom of Crystal Chair there is a cat track that leads away from the lift towards the Blackcomb Glacier Rescue Road. Three hundred metres down the track on the left is a short sidestep up to a height-of-land. Work your way down and left from this blunt ridge to find a series of cliff drops and lines through the old growth forest. Worth a look!

86 In the Spirit ♦ ★

(No photo – see mountain map) From the bottom of the Crystal Chair, this gladed run descends to the Blackcomb Glacier Rescue Road. The pitch is nice but it requires at least two metres of snow to fill in the creeks and cover the downed trees.

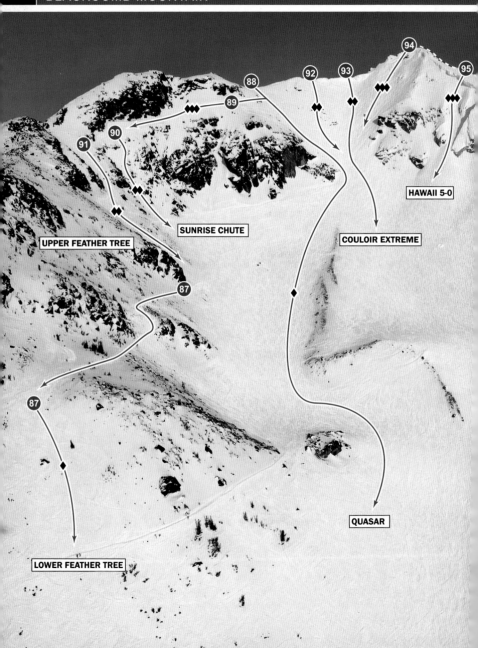

HAWAII 5-0

SUNRISE CHUTE

COULOIR EXTREME

UPPER FEATHER TREE

QUASAR

LOWER FEATHER TREE

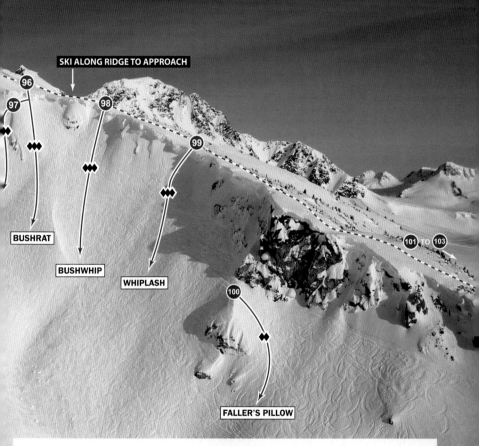

SKI ALONG RIDGE TO APPROACH

96

97

98

99

BUSHRAT

BUSHWHIP

WHIPLASH

101 TO 103

100

FALLER'S PILLOW

⑪ Chainsaw Ridge

The 7th Heaven chairlift is the gateway to Blackcomb's high alpine. With amazing terrain in every direction, the lift allows you to find whatever you're looking for, including Chainsaw Ridge, the showpiece steeps visible from the Rendezvous restaurant and home of the famous Couloir Extreme. Access the top of Chainsaw Ridge via the lookout north of the Horstman Hut restaurant.

㊐ Feather Tree ♦ ★★

Feather Tree is the name given to the slope below the cliffs between Cougar Chutes (Secret Zone) and Quasar. Access can be gained via traverse in from either side.

88 Quasar ♦ ★

The easiest line in the zone. Sneak into the bowl at the farthest-right gate and work the slope on the skiers right of the lateral moraine.

89 Sunrise Traverse ♦♦♦ ★

This run starts on the skier's right of Quasar and crosses above the large cliff to access the slopes on the opposite side of the bowl. Photo on page 152.

90 Sunrise Chute ♦♦ ★

The chute only becomes skiable on big snow seasons when a three-metre-plus snow base covers the rocks. When in shape, it's a nice slide down to the moraine. Photo on page 152.

91 Upper Feather Tree ♦♦ ★★

The furthest chute right past Sunrise, pick your way down to join Feather Tree. Photo on page 152.

92 Big Bang ♦♦ ★

Think of it as the Couloir's little brother. Ski in 15 metres (50 feet) right of the entrance to the Couloir Extreme main chute. Work the terrain left of the rocky moraine in the bowl. Also known as "Sylvan".

93 Couloir Extreme ♦♦ ★★

An ultra-popular mega-couloir. The line is right down the centre of the bowl. Formerly known as

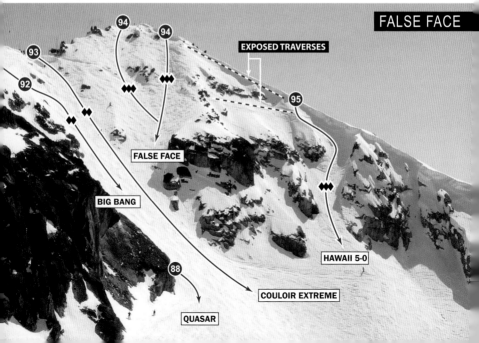

FALSE FACE

EXPOSED TRAVERSES

FALSE FACE

BIG BANG

HAWAII 5-0

COULOIR EXTREME

QUASAR

the Saudan Couloir, this has been the staging place for the thigh-burning horror show known as the Couloir Extreme race.

⑨⑭ False Face ◆◆◆ ★

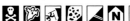

Serious mountain terrain that's not for the faint of heart. This line is one of the steepest skiable faces at any ski area in North America.

⑨⑤ Hawaii 5-0 ◆◆◆ ★★

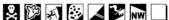

Skiing for the ultra-hardcore. Don't fall!

⑨⑥ Bushrat ◆◆◆ ★★★

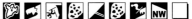

Ski about halfway down the ridge to the obvious notch entrance in the cornice. From here, drop in and ski the diagonal chute.

⑨⑦ Bushrat Shoulder ◆◆◆ ★★

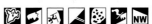

Bushrat Shoulder shares the same entrance as Bushrat proper. Once you are in the bowl, ride the shoulder fall line below the and skier's right of the main chute.

⑨⑧ Bushwhip ◆◆◆ ★★★

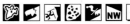

Sandwiched between Bushrat and Whiplash lies Bushwhip. The entrance can be tricky and very dangerous depending on now the cornice forms. Scope if from below first!

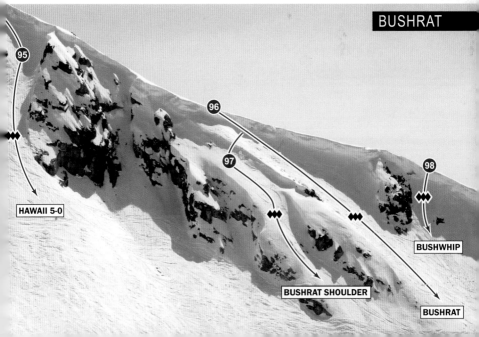

BUSHRAT

HAWAII 5-0

BUSHWHIP

BUSHRAT SHOULDER

BUSHRAT

99 Whiplash ◆◆◆ ★★

Sometimes this line goes and sometimes it doesn't, depending on the cornice. Scope it out from below, before you try to find a way in!

100 Faller's Pillow ◆◆ ★★★

This slope is on the skier's left of the cliffs, in the middle of the bowl. Often the deepest snow in the zone. Bring your snorkel!

101 Regulator ◆◆ ★

The lower third of the ridge starts with this open line. Would-be Whistler extremists should consider this their right of passage. Snowboarders can get that signature cornice 540 shot here!

102 Dog Leg ◆ ★

The crooked line downhill from the Regulator cornice.

103 High Test / Low Test ◆ ★

Two convex rolls at the bottom of the ridge.

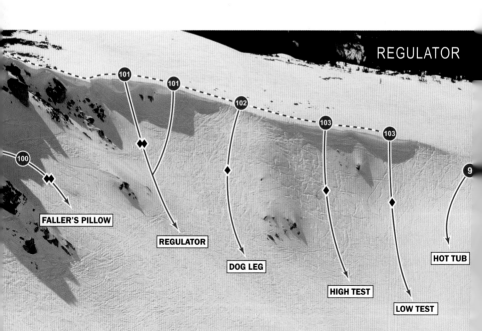

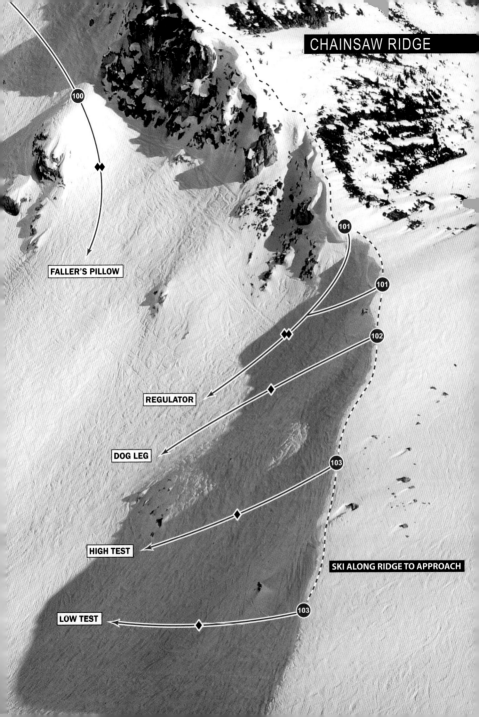

CHAINSAW RIDGE

100

FALLER'S PILLOW

101

101

102

REGULATOR

DOG LEG

103

HIGH TEST

SKI ALONG RIDGE TO APPROACH

LOW TEST

103

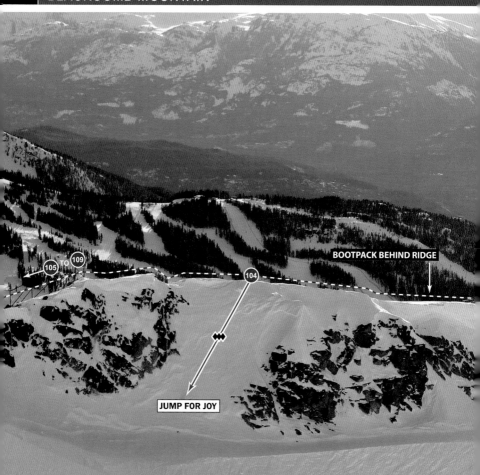

BOOTPACK BEHIND RIDGE

105 TO 109

104

JUMP FOR JOY

Local's Tip

Timing is everything! If you get to the Horstman
Zone early on a powder day, consider doing a few
"short but sweet" laps on the T-bars before dropping
down to the lower lifts and rejoining the masses!
Hey, you beat the crowds, so reap the rewards!

⑫ Horstman Peak

The ridge rising above the 7th Heaven Chair reaches Horstman peak above the Blowhole and Blackcomb Glacier. The lower-angled south side is visible as you ride up the 7th Heaven Chair, and the steeper skiable terrain on the north side is described below. Access is gained by walking behind the top tower of the Horstman T-bar to gain the bootpack onto the ridge.

⑩ Jump For Joy ◆◆◆ ★★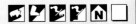

The first skiable face that you get to on the ridge. Short and steep. If you feel sketchy, just think about the guy who successfully rode his mountain bike down this for a Warren Miller movie!

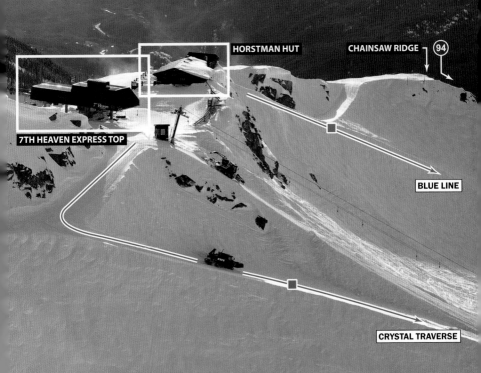

HORSTMAN HUT

CHAINSAW RIDGE ⑭

7TH HEAVEN EXPRESS TOP

BLUE LINE

CRYSTAL TRAVERSE

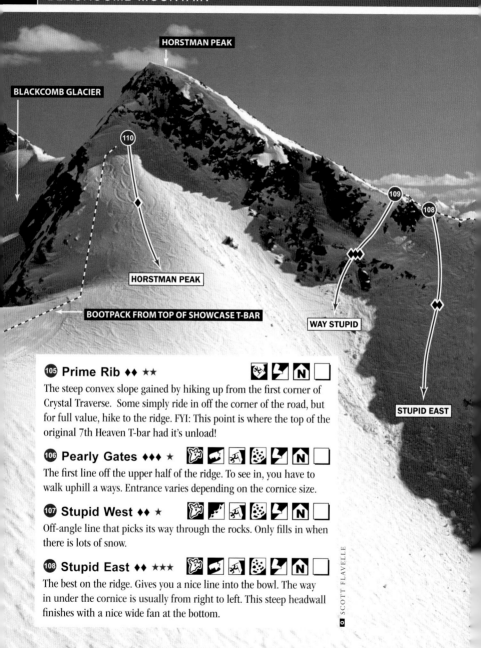

HORSTMAN PEAK

BLACKCOMB GLACIER

110

109

108

HORSTMAN PEAK

BOOTPACK FROM TOP OF SHOWCASE T-BAR

WAY STUPID

STUPID EAST

© SCOTT FLAVELLE

105 Prime Rib ♦♦ ★★

The steep convex slope gained by hiking up from the first corner of Crystal Traverse. Some simply ride in off the corner of the road, but for full value, hike to the ridge. FYI: This point is where the top of the original 7th Heaven T-bar had it's unload!

106 Pearly Gates ♦♦♦ ★

The first line off the upper half of the ridge. To see in, you have to walk uphill a ways. Entrance varies depending on the cornice size.

107 Stupid West ♦♦ ★

Off-angle line that picks its way through the rocks. Only fills in when there is lots of snow.

108 Stupid East ♦♦ ★★★

The best on the ridge. Gives you a nice line into the bowl. The way in under the cornice is usually from right to left. This steep headwall finishes with a nice wide fan at the bottom.

109 Way Stupid ♦♦♦ ★

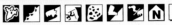

This chute is only skiable in the fattest conditions. The problem is that when conditions are fat, so is the cornice! Most people traverse in from Stupid East.

110 Horstman Peak ♦ ★

This slope is the big powder fan that builds up under the north face of the Peak. Access is gained by riding the Showcase T-bar, traversing over and bootpacking up the fan.

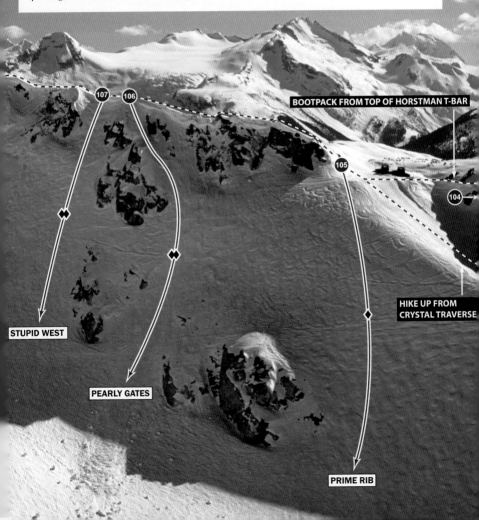

BOOTPACK FROM TOP OF HORSTMAN T-BAR

STUPID WEST

PEARLY GATES

HIKE UP FROM
CRYSTAL TRAVERSE

PRIME RIB

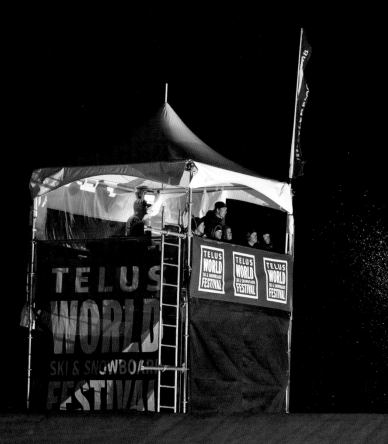

The Big Air competition at the World Ski and Snowboard Festival is one of Whistler's key attractions.

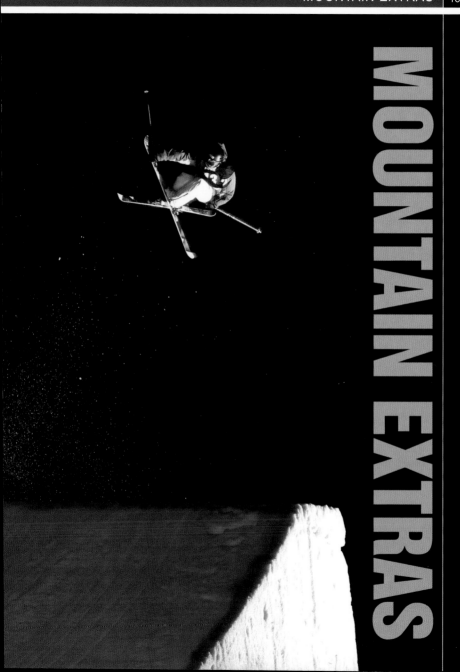

MOUNTAIN EXTRAS

Terrain Parks

There's no debating the fact that terrain park skiing and riding has come of age in the second decade of the new millennium. What was considered a distant afterthought to downhill racing a mere ten years ago has developed into the main attraction for the young generation. The rise of snowboard pipe as one of the most watched events at the 2010 Olympics (second only to the gold medal round of men's hockey) and the acceptance of skier pipe into the 2014 Games has catapulted those that stand atop the podiums to rock star status. Slopestyle will inevitably join the fold and when combined with pipe and snowcross the trilogy of terrain park disciplines will be complete. There is little doubt that the kids riding the parks of today are destined to be the most revered Olympians of tomorrow.

Whistler Blackcomb has dedicated a talented and qualified crew to create and maintain their terrain parks. One of the chief priorities of the parks team is to continuously provide a cutting edge product for riders of all ability levels. As a result, the resort has received over 30 top ten awards for innovation and design.

The parks at Whistler Blackcomb are designed to allow a progression of skills with jumps ranging from 1.5–27 metres (5–90 feet) as well as boxes, rails, half-pipes and Canada's only permanent snowcross track open for public riding.

If you are new to the park-riding scene there's a few survival tips that are crucial to learn. These tips are aligned with an unwritten code of conduct that has roots in both surf and skateboard etiquette.

❑ Take a lesson if you're new to the sport.

❑ Ski / ride features that are appropriate to your ability level. Overreaching your skill level makes you a hazard to yourself and others.

❑ Before dropping in to a feature call out "Dropping in", to signal your intent.

❑ Clear the landing area as quickly as possible after you land (or crash).

❑ Stop only in a safe place where you are visible to riders above.

❑ Dropping in before your turn (snaking) is generally not accepted unless you are by far the best rider in the park! As with all session sports, a pecking order is established and must be respected.

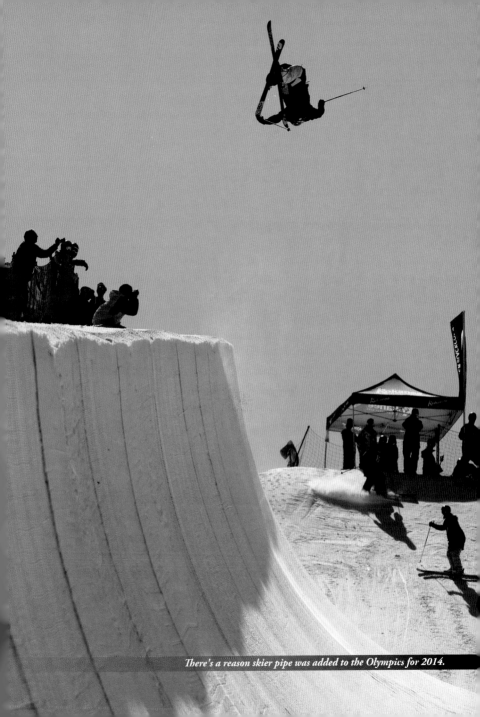

There's a reason skier pipe was added to the Olympics for 2014.

Whistler Terrain Parks

Whistler has two excellent parks that appeal to the novice and intermediate park user. Both are accessed off the Emerald Express chairlift.

❶ Cougar Terrain Park ★★★

This is Whistler's mini park and features small and extra-small jumps and rail features. Cougar Park breaks off left after the entrance gate above the Peak 2 Peak tower. It's a great spot for new park riders to learn basic tricks.

❷ Chipmunk Terrain Park ★★★

The main park on the Whistler side. This mid-level park has multiple lines offering features for the average rider. In many ways, "Chippy" has the best slope angle for park building and allows for creative rail combinations and jump rhythm sections. As a result it is a very popular park that can attract significant crowds on sunny days. This zone includes both the Green Acres and Bobcat terrain parks.

Follow this mantra daily for the best park riding experience: "Preride, Reride, Freeride"

Preride – Slide through the park and look at the features. Remember, they get rebuilt and changed everyday. Use this lap to assess which features are appropriate for you skill level.

Reride – Ride through the park a second time, checking the speed of your gear and the snow. Ride up the take-offs and see what kind of transitions they have. Try and gauge how much speed you'll need to clear them.

Freeride – With two warm-up laps down, you should be good to go, but remember to ride with care!

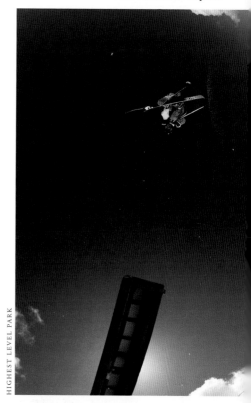

HIGHEST LEVEL PARK

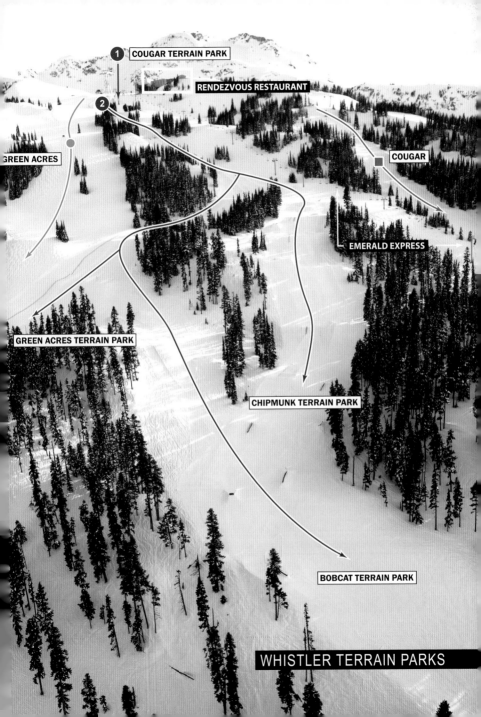

1 COUGAR TERRAIN PARK

RENDEZVOUS RESTAURANT

COUGAR

2

GREEN ACRES

EMERALD EXPRESS

GREEN ACRES TERRAIN PARK

CHIPMUNK TERRAIN PARK

BOBCAT TERRAIN PARK

WHISTLER TERRAIN PARKS

Blackcomb Terrain Parks

Blackcomb has a full selection of terrain parks for all users from beginner through world-class expert.

❸ Big Easy Terrain Garden ★★★

Located on Blackcomb off Easy Out, "The Garden" offers even the first-time park rider a chance to session freestyle terrain features. This area has, jumps, rollers, banks and boxes to get your feet wet. Access is via the Solar Coaster Express chair.

❹ Nintendo Choker Terrain Park ★★

The entrance to the Choker Park aka "Blue Park" lies between the top of Solar Coaster and the top of Catskinner. The mix in this park includes a range of medium to large features with the focus on skill development and creative use of the terrain for rails. A small, five-metre mini-pipe is often built on this run when snow volume allows.

❺ The Highest Level ★★★

Contained within the Nintendo Park is the Highest Level (HL) or "Black Park". This zone offers the largest snow features in the world open for public use! A special park pass is required for access. Users must sign a waiver to obtain the pass (available at Guest Relations) and wear a helmet at all times. This is the home of the "Shack Booter", "Tower Hit" and "Kong", which grows to over 27 metres (90 feet) annually. The HL is where the sport is being pushed ever further into the future as athletes conjure spins that boggle the mind. To view all the action from above, ride the Catskinner chair!

On days when there is a lot of new snow, an entity known as the "Powder Park" is created within the confines of the HL. Since the high speeds required to hit the features in the park are impossible when blanketed by new snow, the jumps remain closed until the grooming machines can catch up. Highest Level pass holders can still flash their passes and get an exclusive powder shred behind the ropes. There is even a crew of grey haired locals that finagle HL passes for just such occasions and never hit a single jump in the park!

❻ Global Superpipe ★★★

This monster half-pipe can be found at the bottom of the Nintendo Park on the right side. Cut nightly with the Global Pipe Shaper, the seven-metre transition walls are of Olympic standard. Pipes cut to this size are a requirement for the triple cork aerials that are winning the contests of today.

❼ Snowcross ★★★

For the uninitiated, a Snowcross course is the mountain version of motor-cross complete with berms, corners, jumps and whoop-de-dos. In competitions like the Olympics and X-Games, racers match up four at a time for an all out race to the bottom. Recreationally, the course is fun for showdowns between friends or even a solo cruise. Access to the course is through a gate on the left side of Springboard under the Solar Coaster Express.

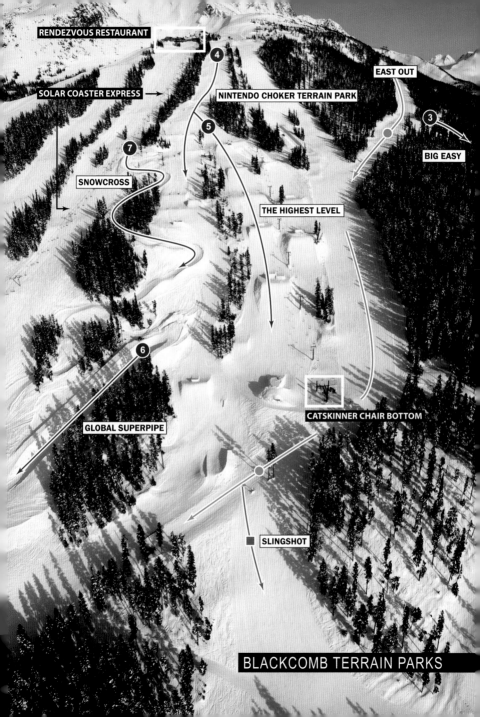

BLACKCOMB TERRAIN PARKS

Link-ups

The best way to get the most value out of each run on the hill is to link a few lines together and make an epic descent out of it. Try these to start; you'll soon develop a list of your own!

BLACKCOMB

From Showcase T-Bar:

☐ Blowhole—Surf's Up

☐ Blowhole—Winky Pop

☐ Ladies First—Husume Flank

From Spanky's Ladder:

☐ Diamond Left—Calvin—Hobbes

☐ Emerald Bowl—Zut Zut

☐ Spanky's Chute—Playland

☐ Spanky's Chute—Shredder

☐ Spanky's Shoulder—Playland

☐ Blackcomb Bowl:

☐ Couloir Extreme—Faller's Pillow

☐ Bushrat—Faller's Pillow

☐ Big Bang—Blowdown

☐ Quasar—Staircase

From Solar Coaster Express:

☐ Bark Sandwich—Little Cub

WHISTLER

From the Peak Express:

☐ Whistler Bowl—Doom and Gloom—Grande Finale

☐ Whistler Bowl—Sunrise (or Escalator)—Grande Finale

☐ West Cirque—Everglades—Peak to Creek

☐ West Cirque—Frog Hollow

☐ Whistler Bowl—Surprise

☐ Whistler Bowl—Shale Slope

☐ Whistler Bowl—Tiger's Terrace

From the Harmony Express:

☐ Little Whistler—Camel Backs—Bitter End—Boot Chutes

☐ Harmony Horseshoe 5—Boomer Bowl—Wet Dreams

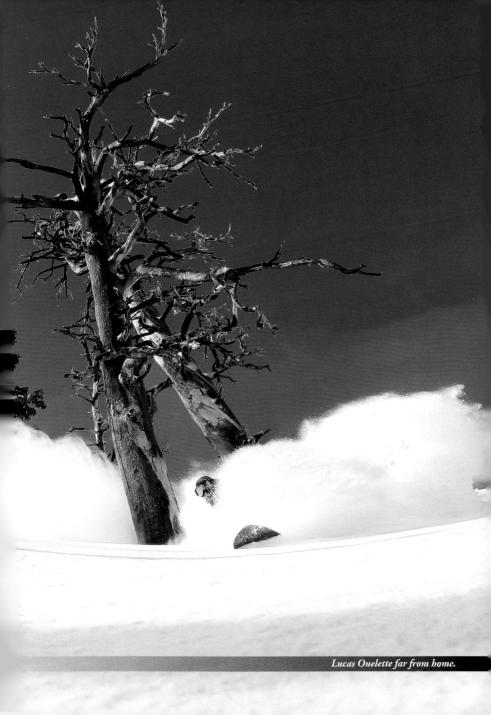

Lucas Ouelette far from home.

The Groomed Runs

As the marketing department is apt to remind you, Whistler Blackcomb has some of the best cat drivers in the industry and every night they groom 1,200 to 1,400 acres of terrain. By all accounts, this is more than any other ski resort in North America, and it's the reason we recommend mixing in a few of the classic cruising runs into your daily plan. If you get to them early, you may find 10 centimetres of new snow on top of smooth soft-pack! Here is a list of our favourite groomed runs, all of which are labeled on the trail map:

BLACKCOMB

7th Heaven

- ☐ Cloud Nine
- ☐ Panorama
- ☐ Hugh's Heaven

Crystal Chair

- ☐ Ridge Runner
- ☐ Twist and Shout
- ☐ Rock 'n' Roll

Solar Coaster Express

- ☐ Honeycomb
- ☐ Cruiser
- ☐ Gandy Dancer

Jersey Cream Express

- ☐ Jersey Cream
- ☐ Cougar Milk
- ☐ Zig Zag

WHISTLER

Emerald/Big Red Express

- ☐ Upper and Lower Franz's
- ☐ Upper & Lower Dave Murray Downhill
- ☐ Little Red Run
- ☐ Ptarmigan
- ☐ G.S.
- ☐ Bear Paw

T-Bars

- ☐ T-Bar Run
- ☐ Harmony Piste

Peak Express

- ☐ The Saddle
- ☐ Peak to Creek

Symphony Express

- ☐ Jeff's Ode to Joy
- ☐ Adagio

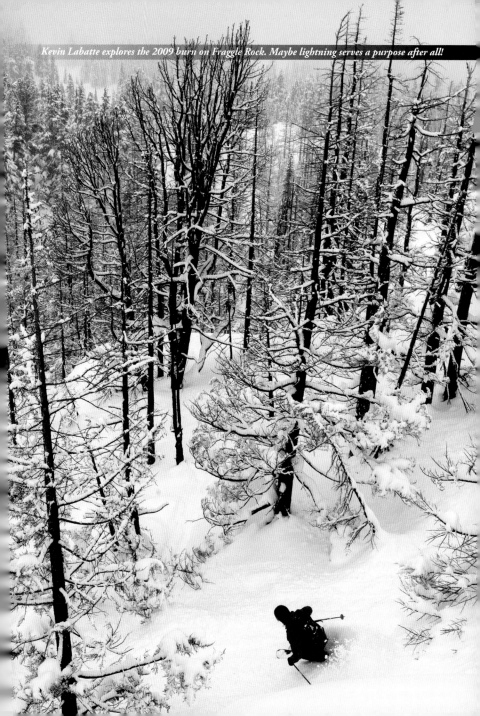

Kevin Labatte explores the 2009 burn on Fraggle Rock. Maybe lightning serves a purpose after all!

Don't Miss List

If you've got limited time or limited attention, here is your hit list. Consider it the best of the best:

BLACKCOMB

- ☐ Blowhole—Surf's Up
- ☐ Ladies First—Husume Flank
- ☐ Sapphire Bowl—Zut Zut
- ☐ Wild Thing—Midbowl Gully
- ☐ Spanky's Chute—Midway Right— Playland
- ☐ Pakalolo Pillow—The Bite
- ☐ Secret Bowl—Dakine
- ☐ Smoked Salmon
- ☐ Couloir Extreme—Coyote Road— Baggers—Bite
- ☐ False Face—Feather Tree
- ☐ Bushrat—Faller's Pillow
- ☐ Bushrat Shoulder—high traverse out at Hot Tub—Glades off 7th Ave
- ☐ Heart Throb—Sluiceway (on trail map)

WHISTLER

- ☐ Excitation
- ☐ The Couloir
- ☐ Whistler Bowl—Shale Slope
- ☐ West Cirque—Sunrise—Grande Finale
- ☐ Stefan's Chute—West Bowl
- ☐ Harmony Ridge—Boomer Bowl— Wet Dreams
- ☐ Pig's Fancy
- ☐ Little Whistler—Camel Back—Boot Chutes
- ☐ McConkey's
- ☐ Sun Bowl—Crescendo
- ☐ Harmony Ridge—Harvey's Harrow
- ☐ T-Bar Run—Old Man—Franz's to the valley

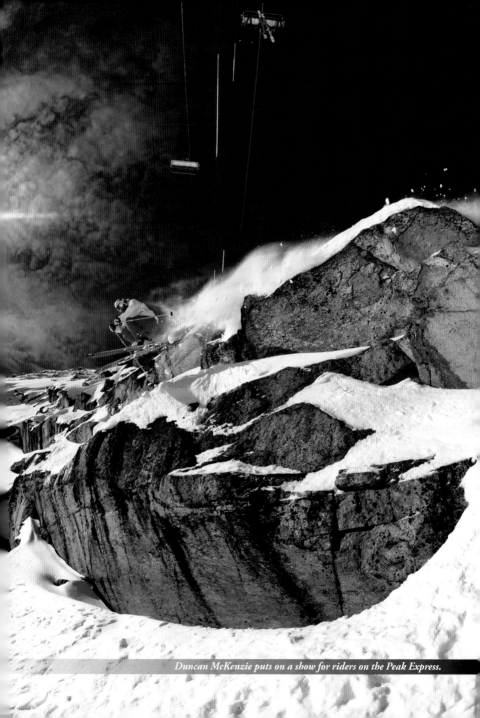

Duncan McKenzie puts on a show for riders on the Peak Express.

Events

Plain and simple, Whistler Blackcomb delivers world-class events. A full-time event staff and an army of volunteers exist behind the scenes working to bring everything from small grassroots races to large-scale week-long festivals. The events calendar fills every season, but the most notable happenings are below. For further details, check Whistlerblackcomb.com

Weekly

Fire & Ice Show: An awesome demonstration of freestyle skills set beside a wicked light show. Seeing the athletes jump through the flaming hoop is always a crowd favorite!

Monthly

The King of the Rail: A jam-format grassroots rail contest held in the Village at the base of Whistler. The setups change monthly, and riders ante up some serious tricks for a shot at the crown.

January

Deep Winter Experience: A week-long celebration of all things winter. Regular events include clinics, camps and demos. The crown jewel of the week is the Deep Winter Photo Challenge in which professional photographers shoot in bounds at Whistler Blackcomb for three days before showing their slideshow to a live audience and panel of judges. The show is a very hot ticket so plan ahead!

February

Peak to Valley Race: This classic giant slalom is a thigh-burning descent from the top of the Saddle on Whistler Mountain to the Creekside base via the Dave Murray Downhill. The after-party is legendary, and most attendees would be hard-pressed to tell you their times, never mind who won.

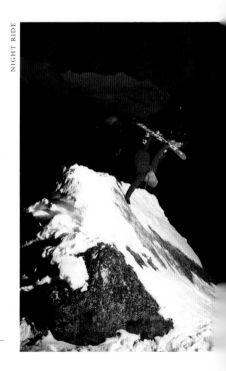

NIGHT RIDE

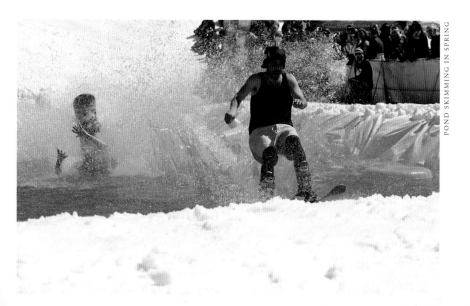

POND SKIMMING IN SPRING

March

Whistler Cup: The most important race in North America for kids age 11 to 14. Athletes from 25 countries compete on the same course on which the Olympians raced in 2010. The podium chasers of tomorrow always impress the spectators.

April

The World Ski and Snowboard Festival: A ten-day celebration of sport, arts and mountain culture that marks the end of winter and the onset of spring. Contests include snowboard halfpipe, slopestyle, big air and custom mixes like the border-style, which combines snowcross racing with jump and style-point elements. The prize purses are large so the best skiers in the world come to compete.

May

Crud to Mud: The final race of the winter calendar coincides with the start of the mountain biking season. Racers tackle a G.S. course from the Roundhouse on Whistler Mountain to the bottom of Garbanzo Express. At Garbanzo, they shed their ski and snowboard gear, symbolizing the end of winter, and transition to mountain bikes on which they continue to race to the valley.

Index of Runs by Name

A
Adagio 72
Arthur's Choice 148

B
Bad Attitude 134
Bagel Bowl 99
Bagel Roll 98
Bagger 1 119
Bagger 2 119
Bagger 3 119
Bernie's Bumps 99
Big Bang 154
Big Easy Terrain Garden 168
Big Timber 102
Bite, The 119
Bitter End 56
Blowdown 119
Blowhole, The 124
Bonsai 95
Boomer Bowl 55
Boot Chutes 54
Bushrat 155
Bushrat Shoulder 155
Bushwhip 155

C
Café Chute 117
Calvin 134
Camel Backs 58
CBC 148
C.C. 40
Chipmunk Terrain Park 166
Chris's Drop 88

Chunky's Choice 44
Circle Chute 138
Cirque, The 82
Clean Out 138
Club 21 48
Cockalorum 96
Come Chute 91
Cougar Chutes 142
Cougar Terrain Park 166
Couloir Extreme 154
Couloir, The 82
Crack House 125
Cream Cheese Ridge 98
Crystal Glide Cliffs 151
Curl, The 141

D
Dakine 145
Danger Bay 146
Dapper's Delight 44
Davies Dervish 145
Diamond Bowl 134
Die Hard 56
Dilemma 58
Dog Leg 156
Don't Stop 145
Doom and Gloom 86
Dusty's Descent 102

E
Easy Route 77
Elevator 92
Encore Ridge 81
Escalator 92
Everglades 95
Excitation 58
Exhilaration 58

F

Faller's Pillow 156
False Face 155
Family Jewels 132
Feather Tree 153
Flute Main Bowl 78
Flute North Bowl 78
Flute Shoulder 78
Fraggle Rock 150
Franz's Meadow 38
Frog Hollow 92
Front Page Challenge 147

G

Garbanzo Lift Line 46
Garnet Bowl 131
Glacier Wall 58
Glissando Glades 74
Global Superpipe 168
Goat's Gully 42
Grande Finale 86
Grey Zone, The 146
G.S. Start 53
Gummy Bear 136
Gun Barrels 55

H

Haole Rock 145
Harmony Ridge 60
Harvey's Harrow 67
Hawaii 5-0 155
Headwall 52
Heartthrob 121
Heavenly Basin 145
Hidden Chute 67
Highest Level, The 168
High Test / Low Test 156

Hobbes 134
Home Run 102
Horseshoe 1 61
Horseshoe 3 61
Horseshoe 4 61
Horseshoe 5 61
Horseshoe 6 60
Horseshoe 7 60
Horseshoe 8 60
Horstman Peak 161
Hot Tub 116
Hourglass 66
Husume Flank 126

I

I.D. Low 121
In Deep 50
Insanity 42
In the Spirit 151

J

Jacob's Ladder 58
Java 124
Jeff's Ode to Joy 72
Jersey Cream Wall 117
Jimmy's Joker 40
Jump For Joy 159
Jump Hill 53

K

Kaleidoscope 62
KC Roll 62
Key West 90
Krakatoa 125

L

Ladies First 125

Lakeside Centre 120
Left Hook 90
Lesser Flute 81
Lesser Flute Bowl 81
Liftie's Leap 84
Lines off 7th Avenue 112
Little Cub 114
Little Whistler 58
Log Jam 150
Lower McConkey's 54
Lower V.D. Chutes 38
Low Roll 62
Lox Chute 98
Luger's Run 114

M
Mid-Bowl Roll/Gully 134
Midway Rock 136
Molly's Reach 146
Monday's 96
Moraine 78
My Line 138

N
Nintendo Choker Terrain Park 168
North Bowl Cornice 80
North Chute 78
North Face Low 88

O
Outer Limits 148
Overbite 145

P
Pacer Chute 86
Pacer Face 86
Pakalolo 142

Pakalolo Pillow 142
Paleface 40
Palooka 68
Peak to Creek 101
Pearly Gates 160
Piccolo Main 72
Piccolo North Face 70
Pig's Fancy 78
Pipeline 141
Playland 136
Prime Rib 160
Pumphouse Roll 117
Purple Haze 142

Q
Quasar 154

R
Raptors Ride 113
Ratfink 44
Regulator 156
Renegade Glade 114
Rhapsody Bowl 74
Rider's Revenge 150
Robertson's Run 67
Roger's Rush 54
Romper Room 147
Rumble in the Trunks 68

S
Saddle, The 82
Safe Route 62
Safe Route Chutes 66
Salmon Belly 145
Sapphire Bowl 132
Sapphire Chutes 132
Secret Bowl 140

Secret Chute 140
Seppo's 46
Shale Chute 90
Shale Slope 88
Shredder 136
Side Order 49
Skid Lips 136
Smoked Salmon 145
Sneaky Pete 95
Snowcross 168
Spanky's Chute 136
Spanky's Ladder 128
Spanky's Shoulder 136
Spoon, The 117
Staccato Glades 74
Staggerhome Chute 53
Staircase 119
Stefan's Chute 98
Stuie's Slope 78
Stupid East 160
Stupid West 160
Summit Slope 70
Sun Bowl 66
Sun Bowl Chutes 66
Sunrise 92
Sunrise Chute 154
Sunrise Traverse 154
Surf's Up 132
Surprise 88
Swiss Cheese 138

T

T-Bar Bowl 52
Teetering 142
Tiger's Terrace 90
Traverse Pillow 120
Tree Fall 117

U

Unsanctioned 50
Upper Feather Tree 154
Upper V.D. Chutes 90

W

Watch Out 113
Waterface 56
Way Stupid 161
West Cirque 86
Wet Dreams 55
Where's Joe 113
Whiplash 156
Whistler Cornice 84
Whistler Bowl Main Entrance 84
Whistler Village Gondola Lift Line . . . 46
Wildcard 40
Wild Thing 134
Wind Lip, The 122
Winky Pop 132

Y

Yard Sale 113

Z

Zudrell's 44
Zut Zut 132

MOONRISE ABOVE 7TH HEAVEN

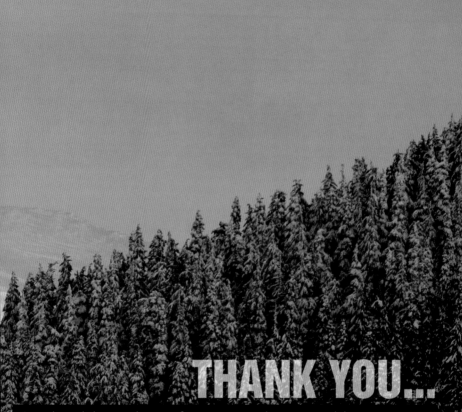

THANK YOU...

Several people have made a significant impact on this project and deserve our gratitude. We would like to thank the following:

Our publisher and friend Marc Bourdon for his constant willingness to embrace our ideas and for always pushing us toward the creation of an exceptional product. Shawn Beaudoin and Nigel Stewart for their meticulous proofreading. Ian Hodder for editing our manuscript and not making fun of our atrocious grammar. Robert Kennedy for his words of advice and encouragement. Brian Leighton and Ian Bunbury for providing insight that can only come from decades spent on the hill. And of course, our families for supporting our project and giving us a few spare moments at the computer or behind the camera! Thank you all very much, we sincerely appreciate it!

Brian Finestone has worked for Whistler Blackcomb for twenty years in virtually every role in the operations division, from parks to patrol to management. Despite the thousands of days he has spent on the hill he still frequents the bowls and parks while passing on his passion for skiing and riding to his son. After catching the writing bug with the first edition

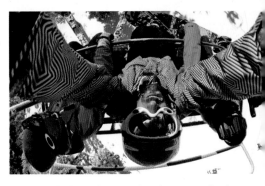

of the Ski and Snowboard Guide to Whistler Blackcomb, Brian has become a freelance writer and photographer in his spare time with articles published around the world on snow sports, surfing and biking adventures. Brian continues to live the dream life in Whistler with his wife and son, logging hundreds of days per year on his snowboard, bikes and skis.

Kevin Hodder splits his time between guiding in the mountains and working as a television producer. His career has taken him to some of the most beautiful places in the world but he has always returned to Whistler where he lives with his wife and young daughter. Kevin's passions involve all things that Whistler is famous for including mountain biking, climbing, hiking, trail running, road biking and, of course, skiing!

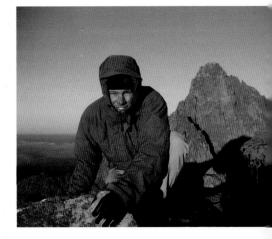